MEDICAL ASPECTS OF DEVELOPMENTAL DISABILITIES IN CHILDREN BIRTH TO THREE

REVISED FIRST EDITION

Editor
James A. Blackman, M.D.

Assistant Professor
Department of Pediatrics
College of Medicine
The University of Iowa

Pediatrician, Infant and Young Child Service
Department of Pediatrics
University Hospital School
The University of Iowa Hospitals and Clinics
Iowa City, Iowa

AN ASPEN PUBLICATION ®

Aspen Systems Corporation
Rockville, Maryland
Royal Tunbridge Wells
1984

Library of Congress Cataloging in Publication Data
Main entry under title:

Medical aspects of developmental disabilities in
children birth to three.

"An Aspen publication."
Includes index.
1. Developmentally disabled children. 2. Children—Diseases.
I. Blackman, James A. [DNLM: 1. Child Development Disorders.
2. Child Development Disorders—diagnosis.
3. Health Status. WS 350.6 M489]
RJ135.M43   1984   618.92   84-11128
ISBN: 0-89443-553-1

Publisher: John Marozsan
Associate Publisher: Jack W. Knowles, Jr.
Editorial Director: Margaret Quinlin
Executive Managing Editor: Margot G. Raphael
Managing Editor: M. Eileen Higgins
Editorial Services: Scott Ballotin
Printing and Manufacturing: Debbie Collins

Based on a grant from the Division of Maternal Child
Health, Department of Health and Human Services
to the University of Iowa.

Library of Congress Catalog Card Number: 84-11128
ISBN: 0-89443-553-1

Printed in the United States of America

3   4   5

This book is dedicated to infants and young children with special needs and to special-service providers who help meet those needs.

Introduction

The health status of disabled children has a profound effect on their development. It is therefore essential that early intervention professionals in the educational setting are knowledgeable about the health and functioning of the children they serve. Without such knowledge, educators may be unaware of—or they may *overestimate*—the limitations that particular conditions or treatments can place on a child's progress.

Medical records are routinely sought by early education programs, but often these contain jargon understandable only to members of the health profession. The same may be said of textbooks written by and for physicians. Even individuals with training in the health field may have difficulty keeping up with countless new developments in the diagnosis and management of the various conditions. What is needed—and what this manual seeks to provide—is an accessible, easy-to-understand resource on those conditions, tests, and other health care issues that are relevant to infants and young children with developmental disabilities. Topics—arranged alphabetically for ease of reference—were selected on the basis of a survey of professionals who deliver services in early intervention and education programs.

This manual is not a resource for educational and therapeutic techniques. Neither is it an exhaustive treatment of any given topic (for this, the reader may want to consult specialized textbooks, journals, or health care professionals). Rather, it is a summary of that health information which is important to the care of a particular child—with special emphasis on those aspects of a condition which affect day-to-day functioning.

We recommend that this manual be readily available to all professionals—including medical professionals—who work with developmentally disabled children; and we encourage limited duplication of sections applicable to appropriate service providers.

Acknowledgments

The editor wishes to thank Alfred Healy, M.D., Chairman of the Division of Developmental Disabilities, Department of Pediatrics, The University of Iowa, who provided the igniting spark for this manual.

I would also like to express my gratitude to Merle McPherson, M.D., Chief, Habilitative Services Branch, Division for Maternal and Child Health, and to Camille L. Cook, R.N., M.S. Nursing Consultant, DMCH, for their advice and encouragement.

For their review of individual chapters, I am indebted to the following people: From The University of Iowa, Richard C. Ahrens, M.D., Richard Andersen, M.D., James F. Bale, M.D., James A. Bartley, M.D., Edward F. Bell, M.D., William E. Bell, M.D., Robert M. Bumsted, M.D., Marjorie E. Caruth, M.S., R.D., Lynne S. Cobb, Ph.D., Brenda Cruikshank, M.D., James W. Hanson, M.D., Dennis C. Harper, Ph.D., Brian F. McCabe, M.D., Hughlett Morris, Ph.D., William J. Marvin, M.D., Gail A. McGuinness, M.D., Christy L. A. Nelson, O.T.R., Kevin C. Pringle, M.D., William J. Rhead, M.D., Wilbur L. Smith, M.D., Ronald G. Strauss, M.D., Luke Y. Tsai, M.D., Hans U. Zellweger, M.D., William E. Scott, M.D., Stuart L. Weinstein, M.D.; from the Chicago Medical School, C. Murphy Combs, Ph.D.; and from the University of Wisconsin-Madison, Michael G. Block, Ph.D.

Particular thanks go to four individuals who reviewed the manual in its entirety and offered detailed suggestions for its improvement. They are Kathryn E. Barnard, Ph.D., University of Washington; Suzann K. Campbell, Ph.D., University of North Carolina; Alfred L. Scherzer, Ed.D., M.D., The New York Hospital-Cornell Medical Center; and Margaret G. Weiser, Ed.D., The University of Iowa.

I would also like to thank the professionals in the early educational and early intervention programs of Iowa and Kansas for their help, both in selecting topics and in field testing materials for this manual.

Finally, I am grateful to the following individuals for their assistance in the preparation of this manual: research assistant Pamela Hodgman; graphic artists Nancy King, Richard Huber, Rebecca Stutts Connor, and Richard McAfee; and typists Karn Reinke and Karla Johannesen.

Special thanks goes to the assistant editor, Marilyn Knight, for her competence and commitment in coordinating this project and in organizing and refining the content of this book.

Contributors

Blackman, James A., M.D.
Assistant Professor
Department of Pediatrics
College of Medicine
The University of Iowa

Pediatrician, Infant and Young Child Service
Division of Developmental Disabilities
The University of Iowa Hospitals and Clinics
Iowa City, Iowa

Hardy, James C., Ph.D.
Professor
Department of Pediatrics
College of Medicine and
Department of Speech Pathology and Audiology
College of Liberal Arts
The University of Iowa

Director of Professional Services
Division of Developmental Disabilities
The University of Iowa Hospitals and Clinics
Iowa City, Iowa

Healy, Alfred, M.D.
Professor
Department of Pediatrics
College of Medicine and
Division of Special Education
College of Education
The University of Iowa

Chairman
Division of Developmental Disabilities
The University of Iowa Hospitals and Clinics
Iowa City, Iowa

Henderson, Marcia, R.N., M.A., C.P.N.P.
Pediatric Nurse Practitioner
Division of General Pediatrics
Children's Hospital of Los Angeles
Los Angeles, California

Kahn, Gerri, Ph.D., CCC-A
Audiologist
Division of Developmental Disabilities
The University of Iowa Hospitals and Clinics
Iowa City, Iowa

Lough, Loretta Knutson, L.P.T., M.A.
Adjunct Associate Faculty
Physical Therapy Education
The University of Iowa
Iowa City, Iowa

Senior Physical Therapist
Division of Developmental Disabilities
The University of Iowa Hospitals and Clinics

Mapel, Janet R., R.N., B.S.N., C.P.N.P.
Pediatric Nurse Practitioner
Child and Young Adult Service
Division of Developmental Disabilities
The University of Iowa Hospitals and Clinics
Iowa City, Iowa

Nowak, Arthur J., D.M.D.
Professor
Department of Pedodontics
College of Dentistry
The University of Iowa

Supervisor of Dental Services
Division of Developmental Disabilities
The University of Iowa Hospitals and Clinics

Director
Division of Pedodontics
Department of Hospital Dentistry
The University of Iowa Hospitals and Clinics
Iowa City, Iowa

Schor, David P., M.D.
Assistant Professor
Department of Pediatrics
College of Medicine
The University of Iowa

Pediatrician
Child Development Clinic
Division of Developmental Disabilities
The University of Iowa Hospitals and Clinics
Iowa City, Iowa

Schultz, Frederick R., M.D.
Assistant Professor
Department of Pediatrics
College of Medicine
The University of Iowa

Pediatrician, PKU and Weight Management Clinics
Division of Developmental Disabilities
The University of Iowa Hospitals and Clinics
Iowa City, Iowa

Solomons, Gerald, M.D.
Professor
Department of Pediatrics
College of Medicine
The University of Iowa

Pediatrician
Child Development Clinic
Division of Developmental Disabilities
The University of Iowa Hospitals and Clinics

Acting Director
Institute of Child Behavior and Development
The University of Iowa

Codirector, Region VII
Children, Youth, and Families
Resource Center
Iowa City, Iowa

Thomson, Elizabeth, J., R.N., M.S.
Clinical Coordinator
Regional Genetic Consultation Service
Division of Medical Genetics
Department of Pediatrics·
The University of Iowa Hospitals and Clinics
Iowa City, Iowa

Wolraich, Mark L., M.D.
Associate Professor
Department of Pediatrics
College of Medicine
The University of Iowa

Pediatrician, Myelodysplastic Clinic
Division of Developmental Disabilities
The University of Iowa Hospitals and Clinics
Iowa City, Iowa

Table of Contents

Anemia

Alfred Healy, M.D.

DESCRIPTION

Anemia is a condition in which the blood is deficient in either red blood cells (RBCs) or hemoglobin, the oxygen-carrying pigment in RBCs.

CAUSE

Anemia occurs when **(1)** there is inadequate production of either red blood cells or hemoglobin or **(2)** when the red blood cells are destroyed or lost faster than they can be replaced.

Inadequate production of either red blood cells or hemoglobin

The production of RBCs or hemoglobin in the bone marrow may be adversely affected by congenital defects which impede the normal division and development of immature cells; by a lack of essential nutrients; or by lead poisoning, drugs, infection, malignancy, irradiation, kidney disease, or any chronic debilitating condition. The most common cause, however, is iron deficiency.

Iron-deficiency anemia results from insufficient daily intake of iron or from excess losses of this mineral through bleeding. A full-term infant is born with enough iron in its body to last only a few months; a premature infant has even less. To accommodate rapid growth, there must be adequate iron in the diet. Iron-deficiency anemia may occur in the infant who drinks only breast milk for a prolonged period or in one who drinks a commercial baby formula that is not iron-fortified. It may also occur in the toddler who drinks large quantities of whole milk (low in iron) in lieu of other, iron-rich foods or in the "picky eater" whose food selection excludes iron-rich foods.

At high risk for iron-deficiency anemia are infants with developmental disabilities. The difficulty these children often have with chewing and swallowing disrupts the normal shift from milk to various solid baby foods to table foods—a sequence which usually ensures adequate iron even when there is no awareness of proper nutrition.

Iron-deficiency anemia occurs most often between 9 and 24 months in full-term infants, earlier in those who are premature.

Excessive loss or destruction of red blood cells

Even when the rate of production is normal, red blood cells may be lost or broken down faster than the body can replace them. Normally, an RBC lives for about 120 days before it is replaced by a new RBC, which is made in the bone marrow. In a healthy child or adult, about 1 percent of all RBCs are replaced daily. When the loss or destruction exceeds 1 percent, the bone marrow speeds up production.

Excessive numbers of red blood cells may be lost through hemorrhaging due to surgery, injury, or parasitic infestations in the gastrointestinal tract. Also, RBCs may break down too rapidly because of abnormalities in their enzymes or membranes or because they have deficient or defective hemoglobin. A common anemia caused by defective hemoglobin is sickle cell disease.

Sickle cell disease is transmitted through autosomal recessive inheritance. That is, both parents must be carriers of a gene responsible for abnormal hemoglobin synthesis, and both must pass the gene on to the child. Eight percent of all American Blacks are carriers for sickle cell anemia. When both parents are carriers, there is a 25 percent chance that the offspring will inherit the disease.

Carriers themselves have no difficulty with sickle cell anemia. However, in a person who has the disease, the RBC has a tendency to assume abnormal shapes, becoming long and thin like a sickle instead of round and concave. The sickled RBCs clog blood vessels and fail to circulate and deliver oxygen to the tissues. When this occurs, affected children are severely limited in their activities; too, they are often in considerable pain and very susceptible to certain serious bacterial infections.

CLASSIFICATION OF ANEMIAS BY CAUSE

Anemias caused by inadequate production of red blood cells or hemoglobin:

- Chronic infection or inflammation
- Congenital or acquired aplastic anemias
- Iron deficiency
- Kidney disease
- Lead poisoning
- Malignancy
- Bone marrow damage from irradiation and drugs
- Deficiencies in vitamin B_{12} and folate

Anemias caused by increased destruction or loss of red blood cells:

- Certain drugs
- Hemolytic disease of the newborn
- Immune disorders
- Certain infections
- Sickle cell disease or other hemoglobin disorders
- Certain toxic substances

DETECTION

Anemia can be detected by passing a small sample of blood through a special instrument which automatically detects and records the number of RBCs and amount of hemoglobin therein. Clinics and offices, however, frequently estimate hemoglobin content by filling a small, thin tube with blood and then centrifuging it to separate the RBCs from plasma and other blood elements. The percentage of the total volume occupied by red blood cells (hematocrit) yields an estimate of the amount of hemoglobin in the blood.

Hemoglobin determinations are recommended at nine months (six months for premature infants), then yearly thereafter during routine check-ups. In some localities, it has been the practice to routinely screen for the sickle cell trait among populations with a high incidence of the disease, including Blacks and certain groups with Mediterranean ancestry.

COURSE

Children with mild anemia do not look or act any differently from other children. Children with moderate anemia, however, appear pale and lose the pink coloration of their gums and lips. They also become less active due to the limited amount of oxygen available to burn calories. With severe anemia, heart and breathing rates increase, even at rest. This condition can cause cardiac failure and even—though rarely—death.

A decrease in hemoglobin below expected levels is an excellent indicator of a serious health problem. Detected, such a decrease often prompts remediation of both the anemia and the underlying cause.

With moderate to servere iron-deficiency anemia, increased iron produces notable improvements: in 24 hours there is reduced irritability and increased appetite, and within 72 hours new RBCs are released from the bone marrow. The normal amount of RBCs and hemoglobin are usually attained within one month, but it takes an additional two months to replace the iron stores the infant needs to sustain itself in the event of another period of low iron intake. Supplemental iron is not necessary for all types of anemia; at times it may even be dangerous.

Sickle cell disease is a lifelong condition which may affect longevity. Acute "crises"—characterized by a worsening of the anemia or by pain and swelling of bones, abdominal organs, or other body tissues—may be precipitated by infection or by a reduction of available oxygen; crises may also occur spontaneously for no apparent reason. The most common type is the vaso-occlusive episode, which occurs when abnormally shaped RBCs become trapped in the small blood vessels, depriving tissue of needed oxygen (ischemia) and/or causing the death of small amounts of tissue (infarction). In young children this generally occurs in the bones of the hands and feet. Swelling may also occur around the affected bones. On occasion, sudden, severe anemia may develop, which can be fatal if not treated with intravenous fluids and blood transfusions.

ACCOMPANYING HEALTH PROBLEMS

All types of anemia interfere with the oxygen-carrying capacity of the blood. Therefore, the major effect on the infant is lack of energy to perform the usual developmental tasks of childhood. Iron-deficiency anemia can also cause significant listlessness and irritability. If it is prolonged, it may impede developmental progress.

Sickle cell disease may have associated health disorders, the most important of which is an increased susceptibility to serious, potentially lethal infections. Each child should have an individualized health care plan that is carefully developed by parents and medical professionals.

MEDICAL MANAGEMENT

Once anemia has been discovered, its exact cause should be identified prior to prescribing treatment. Iron-deficiency anemia can be adequately diagnosed and treated by any primary care physician. Other production failure anemias and the hemoglobinopathies, however, may require consultation with a pediatrician or someone specially trained in blood disorders of children (pediatric hematologist).

A well-rounded diet of all the basic food groups provides adequate iron—except during the first year of life, when iron supplementation is recommended. This is most conveniently supplied in an iron-fortified formula for infants, though it can be provided separately. Supplemental iron for exclusively breast-fed infants is usually recommended despite recent evidence suggesting that iron content in breast milk, while low, is very well absorbed by the infant. Any child over a year of age with mild anemia and no other health problems may be treated by dietary changes alone; that way, permanent changes can occur in the child's eating habits.

Consultation regarding iron-deficiency anemia and dietary management is available from dietitians, nutritionists, nurses, or physicians.

IMPLICATIONS FOR EDUCATION

Children with developmental disabilities, both physical and mental, are at high risk for developing iron-deficiency anemia. Education-related professionals can help by encouraging parents to have the child's physician check periodically—and whenever the child is lethargic—for signs of this condition. Educators and therapists can also observe the child for signs of positive response to iron therapy, including increased activity and alertness.

Iron-rich foods should be encouraged—both at home and at school. Offer as many of the following foods as possible each day:
- Meat, fish, or poultry
- Enriched breads and cereals (especially dry baby cereals and cereals fortified with extra iron) and wheat germ
- Dried beans and peas (chili, navy, or pinto beans; split peas)
- Peanut butter
- Dark green, leafy vegetables (spinach, broccoli, chard, kale, beets, turnip greens, dandelion greens)
- Dried fruit (raisins, prunes, dates, figs, apricots)

To help the body utilize the iron content of these foods, offer foods rich in vitamin C at the same time. These include oranges, grapefruit, strawberries, melons, green peppers, and selections from the cabbage family.

Children with or at risk for sickle cell disease should be referred immediately for medical evaluation whenever they have a fever or other signs of an infection. Irritability or lethargy in young children with this disease should be investigated, since these may be symptoms of a sickle cell "crisis."

There has been recent interest in and research on how mild anemia affects learning and development. While results have been equivocal, it is reasonable to assume that a child with optimal health is more likely to benefit from learning experiences. Since moderate to severe (and possibly mild) anemia can influence developmental function and learning, it is important that this condition be recognized, evaluated, and treated promptly.

Approach to Syndromes

Frederick R. Schultz, M.D.

DESCRIPTION

Medical syndromes are various signs and symptoms which occur together commonly enough to warrant giving the pattern a specific name. Down syndrome, for example, is associated with the following characteristics: decreased muscle tone, short stature, a small oral cavity, an upward slant to the eyes, an extra fold at the corner of the eyes, wide spaces between the first and second toes, and short, broad hands with a single palmar crease.

Medical syndromes commonly get their name from the person who first reports the description of the syndrome. Examples include Down, Marfan, and Potter syndromes.

CAUSE

The causes for many syndromes have been identified. It is known, for example, that Down syndrome results from the presence of an extra #21 chromosome. Hurler syndrome results from the absence of the enzyme alpha-L-Iduronidase in the body cells, without which certain substances accumulate in large amounts, causing physical and mental impairment. The physical and mental abnormalities which characterize fetal alcohol syndrome are caused by the effects of alcohol on the brain and other developing organs of the fetus. Finally, Potter syndrome, which is associated with poor lung development, a flat nose, and multicystic kidneys, may occur when there is an unusually small amount of amniotic fluid surrounding the fetus.

The cause of some syndromes is still unknown; an example is Cockayne syndrome, which is associated with poor growth, intellectual impairment, hearing loss, visual impairment, and premature aging.

DETECTION

Most syndromes are diagnosed by observing the abnormalities present and then identifying the pattern. Recognizing a syndrome is important for a number of reasons: it may lead to the identification of potential medical problems, some of which may be treatable; it can also provide parents and educators with information helpful in the planning of individualized instruction or home management. Identifying Waardenburg syndrome, for instance, may lead to the discovery of a hearing loss, which calls for special types of instruction. The identification of certain hereditary syndromes can lead to parental counseling regarding the risks of having another child with the same condition.

Because intellectual limitations characterize many syndromes—Down, William, Noonan, and Prader-Willi, to name a few—it is especially important that children with this disability be examined for signs and symptoms of particular syndromes.

COURSE

Once a particular syndrome is identified, it may be possible to ascertain the likelihood of certain problems developing in the future. Children with Hurler syndrome, for example, should undergo frequent eye and heart examinations, since problems are commonly encountered in these two organs. Children with Prader-Willi syndrome need to have their caloric intake closely monitored because of the rapid and severe obesity which can occur with this condition.

ACCOMPANYING HEALTH PROBLEMS

Serious health problems are a common feature of many medical syndromes. Congenital heart defects, for example, occur frequently with Noonan, Down, Williams, Marfan, and Turner syndromes; kidney abnormalities occur in Turner, Zellweger, and Lowe syndromes. Knowing which health problems are associated with a given syndrome aids in prompt recognition and treatment.

IMPLICATIONS FOR EDUCATION

While certain problems are common with a given syndrome (most children with Down syndrome have intellectual limitations; most with Hurler syndrome have visual, hearing, or cardiac impairments), it is important to keep in mind that *not all children with a particular syndrome are identical.* For example, although most children with Prader-Willi syndrome have intellectual limitations, some do have average abilities. Because a child may have some—but not all—of the features associated with a syndrome, each child must be evaluated individually.

SEE ALSO
Down Syndrome, Fetal Alcohol Syndrome, and *Genetics*

HELPFUL REFERENCES

McKusick, Victor A., M.D. *Mendelian inheritance in man: Catalogs of autosomal dominant, autosomal recessive, and x-linked phenotypes.* Baltimore: The Johns Hopkins University Press, 1978.

Smith, David W., M.D. with Jones, Kenneth Lyons, M.D. *Recognizable patterns of human malformation: Genetic, embryonic, and clinical aspects.* Philadelphia: W. B. Saunders Co., 1982.

Autism

David P. Schor, M.D.

DESCRIPTION

Autism is a developmental disorder with severe distortions of social and language development that begin at an early age. According to the American Psychiatric Association, a child is diagnosed as having infantile autism only if *all* of the following features appear during the first 30 months of life:

- Lack of responsiveness to other people
- Grossly impaired development of language
- Peculiar speech patterns, when speech is present, such as echolalia (repeating the speech of others); pronominal reversal (e.g., the use of "you" for "I"); or metaphorical language (e.g., the repetition of words or sounds with unclear or "private" meanings)
- Bizarre interactions with, or responses to, the environment, such as extreme fascination with unusual objects; resistance to even minor changes; and behavior rituals (often involving repetitive acts such as flicking the fingers) which, if interfered with, lead to great distress or tantrums
- Absence of hallucinations, delusions, and other features of schizophrenia

Children with mental retardation, developmental language disorders, deafness, or childhood schizophrenia may exhibit a few of these features, but their symptoms are generally less severe and more likely to respond to treatment. In very rare cases, the features of autism may not appear until after the first two and one-half years of life. In these instances, however, there is some controversy over whether or not the term *autism* is appropriate.

CAUSE

While autism is thought to be due to brain dysfunction that arises before or around the time of birth, most autistic children do not have a brain injury which is detectable by medical assessments. The prevalence of autism is higher among children with recognized brain injuries, however, than in the population as a whole.

INCIDENCE

Autism is a rare disorder, occurring in about one child in two thousand. It is more common in boys, and the prevalence is significantly increased among siblings of children with autism.

DETECTION

There are no specific laboratory tests that detect autism. The diagnosis is made by observing the child for those features listed above.

The language and social skills of children with autism are not as well developed as their nonverbal cognitive functioning in test or real-life situations. In contrast, the language, social, and cognitive skills of children with mental retardation are all three at similar stages of development.

Careful questioning of parents will usually reveal that the child with autism demonstrated an unusual lack of involvement with others at a very young age. For example, parents may recall lack of eye contact or facial expressiveness in infancy. While some children are reported to have developed relatively normally for up to two years before the onset of symptoms, parental anxiety or lack of knowledge has, in at least some of these cases, masked earlier symptoms.

COURSE

Autism is a chronic disorder; that is, it is manifested at birth (or soon after) and is present throughout the individual's lifetime. While some children are eventually able to lead independent lives after intensive professional services, most continue to require some degree of custodial care. The best predictor of a favorable outcome is the development of useful speech by the age of five.

ACCOMPANYING HEALTH PROBLEMS

Seizures, usually associated with an underlying condition or disease, are rare in the first years yet occur in about 25 percent by early adult life.

MEDICAL MANAGEMENT

No specific medical treatment has proven to be effective with autism. Seizures, if present, are treated with medications, just as they are with children who do not have autism.

IMPLICATIONS FOR EDUCATION

Children who have or are suspected of having autism should be observed carefully for possible problems with seeing or hearing. They almost always require special education—focusing on language and self-help skills—along with a systematic and individualized program aimed at modifying inappropriate behavior and improving interaction with others.

Although the autistic child's speech may be complex—these children may have normal or above-normal rote memories—it is unorganized; and when an adult's response is equally complex, the child is unable to comprehend. Some guidelines for communication: keep it simple and direct; use objects or actions in conjunction with words; emphasize functional language (e.g., have the child ask for something by naming it rather than by pointing); and give the child opportunities to interact with younger children, who have a more comparable level of language development. In managing behavior, include tangible rather than social reinforcers and establish predictable routines regarding the sequence of events, the language and gestures you use, and the components of the physical environment.

Parents of children with autism need access to respite care as well as ongoing contact with available, supportive, knowledgeable personnel. They need, especially, assurance that the autism was not caused by a lack of love or attention on their part.

With autism, good communication among parents, educators, and other professionals is particularly important; not only does it facilitate the child's present learning, but it may also reduce or eliminate typical behavior problems that can stand in the way of future development.

SEE ALSO

Hearing Impairment and *Mental Retardation*

Bracing

Loretta Knutson Lough, L.P.T., M.A.

Braces, also known as orthoses, are generally used to assist the child in standing and walking and to prevent contractures or malalignments of joints. Most typically, braces for standing and walking are worn during the day, and those for preventing loss of motion or poor alignment of joints are worn at night.

If a child needs braces, they will be prescribed by an orthopedic specialist, frequently following consultation with a physical therapist. Prescription is based on a variety of factors, including the type and degree of disability, the child's ability to perform functional skills, and his age and social-intellectual development.

Recent years have brought many advances in orthotics. New materials and new styles are now available. Lighter, more cosmetic plastic molded braces are replacing the conventional metal designs, though factors such as growth, material stress, and skin sensitivity sometimes make metal braces more desirable. Styles and preferences vary across the country and around the world. The devices described in the next few pages are representative of commonly used braces.

THE SWIVEL WALKER

The swivel walker (such as that designed by the Orthotic Research and Locomotor Assessment Unit in the United Kingdom) is a rigid body brace mounted on swiveling feet. It is used to encourage early standing and walking without crutches or a walker. This brace is prescribed primarily for children with high-spinal-level myelomeningocele, who have little or no use of the muscles of the lower extremities and who often have muscle weakness in the trunk.

CHEST PAD — Centered over the lower edge of the breastbone (sternum) to prevent leaning forward

PLASTIC CHUTE — Extends the length of the brace in back; helps maintain good posture and is useful in transfers from wheelchair to brace

KNEE BAR WITH PAD — Centered over the knee caps

BASE AND FOOT PLATE ASSEMBLY — Secures foot placement and provides swivel motion

Swivel Walker

The child can walk without crutches by shifting the body weight from side to side. As weight is shifted to one side, the opposite foot plate rises and rotates forward. Swinging the arms with the weight shift increases speed. While a swivel (pivoting) gait pattern is most common, crutches can be used on uneven surfaces with a swing-to (child swings up to the crutches) or a swing-through (child swings past the crutches) gait pattern.

There are no locks at the hips or knees of the swivel walker; therefore, sitting is not possible. However, one experimental variation of the swivel walker combines the base plate assembly of this brace with a parapodium (described below), which *does* have hip and knee locks. This combination is sometimes used with children who already have parapodiums and are accustomed to being able to sit while in the brace.

THE PARAPODIUM

The Canadian parapodium, a body brace mounted on a platform base, is used for standing and walking with the aid of crutches or a walker. Like the swivel walker, it is worn primarily by children who have high-spinal-level myelomeningocele and, therefore, flaccid or semi-flaccid lower extremities and trunk. Hip and knee locks work simultaneously to allow sitting. (The Rochester, New York, variation of the Canadian parapodium allows independent hip and knee joint operation.)

CHEST PAD — Centered over the lower edge of the breastbone (sternum) to prevent leaning forward

BACK PANEL — Centered across the buttocks, with sides extended to one inch below armpits; helps maintain erect posture

KNEE BAR WITH ETHAFOAM PAD — Centered over the kneecaps

FOOT PLATFORM WITH PLASTIC FOOTMOLDS — Heel guard and Velcro-fastening footstraps secure foot position

Parapodium

The child may first pivot walk with the help of an adult and later be taught to use a walker or crutches to execute a swing-to or swing-through gait pattern. A few children will learn to pivot short distances without the aid of an adult, crutches, or a walker.

THE RECIPROCATING GAIT ORTHOSIS (RGO)

The RGO, a plastic molded brace, was first conceived in Canada and later redesigned at Louisiana State University Medical Center. Like the swivel walker and parapodium, it provides the necessary support for children with high-spinal-level myelomeningocele. (It has also been tried with some success on children who have other muscular or neuromuscular problems.) Unlike the swivel walker and parapodium, the RGO has a cable coupling system connecting two separate leg supports. This allows independent leg motion (reciprocal walking) with a walker or crutches. Other special features of the RGO are the pelvic band design and the composite insert at the ankle.

CHEST STRAP — Fastens at the lower edge of the breastbone (sternum)

CABLES — Attach to the hip joints on either side, providing the mechanical drive for walking; disengaging the cables (by unlocking the latch at each hip joint) allows sitting

PELVIC BAND — Fits low across the buttocks to promote erect posture

KNEE-ANKLE-FOOT ORTHOSES (KAFOs) — Provide total contact leg support

COMPOSITE INSERT — Adds extra reinforcement at the ankle

Reciprocating Gait Orthosis (RGO)

To ambulate, the child shifts the body diagonally forward; the resultant traction in the cables causes the opposite leg to swing forward. Use of the RGO is perhaps best preceded by use of the parapodium and/or the swivel walker.

THE HIP-KNEE-ANKLE-FOOT ORTHOSIS (HKAFO)

The metal HKAFO, as shown below, is comprised of long leg braces with a pelvic band. The HKAFO provides support or control at the major joints of the lower extremities—the hip, knee, ankle, and foot. This brace usually attaches to high-top shoes. It is used for children with a variety of developmental disabilities (including high-spinal-level myelomeningocele and cerebral palsy) to stretch muscles or other soft tissues or to assist in standing and walking.

PELVIC BAND
Fits around the waist

METAL UPRIGHTS WITH DROP LOCKS AT HIP AND KNEE JOINTS

THIGH CUFFS

CALF CUFFS

HIGH-TOP SHOES

Hip-Knee-Ankle-Foot Orthosis (HKAFO)

Various locks and joint designs are prescribed according to individual needs. The knees are usually locked when the child is standing or walking. The child may use a swing-to, swing-through, or reciprocal (one-leg-at-a-time) gait pattern.

KNEE-ANKLE-FOOT ORTHOSES (KAFOs)

KAFOs, also known as long leg braces (without pelvic band), are generally used with children who have less functional impairment than children using HKAFOs. Like HKAFOs, KAFOs are used for stretching as well as for standing or walking.

THIGH CUFF

CALF CUFF

CALF STRAP

ANKLE-FOOT ORTHOSIS (AFO)

ORTHOPEDIC SHOES

METAL KAFO   **PLASTIC KAFO**

Knee-Ankle-Foot Orthoses (KAFOs)

KAFOs may be made of metal or plastic. While plastic braces are lighter and more cosmetic (they are less bulky and can often be worn inside regular shoes), metal braces can be lengthened and adjusted more easily for growth. The physician will determine which is suitable for an individual child. A swing-to, swing-through, or reciprocal gait pattern may be used with these braces.

ANKLE-FOOT ORTHOSES (AFOs)

AFOs, commonly called short leg braces, are used with a child who has muscular control at the hip and knee but not at the ankle.

The metal AFO has an ankle joint which can be adjusted to control the up-and-down motion of the foot; the plastic AFO, on the other hand, is molded in a fixed position, most commonly at a 90° angle. The setting of the ankle joint on either brace can influence motion of the knee joint as well as the ankle. Either brace can be adapted to provide medial-lateral ankle support if needed.

Reciprocal walking with or without crutches or a walker is typical with these braces.

METAL AFO   **PLASTIC AFO**

Ankle-Foot Orthoses (AFOs)

TWISTER CABLES

Twister cables are tightly woven coils in a plastic housing used to control the rotation—either inward or outward—of the legs. (Excess inturning of the legs is common in children with cerebral palsy; outturning is common in children with mid-lumbar-level myelomeningocele.)

Reciprocal walking with or without crutches is typical with these braces.

TWISTER CABLES — Connect a pelvic band to shoes or to short leg braces

Twister Cables with
Pelvic Band and Short Leg Braces

THE BODY SHELL

The total contact body shell is most commonly used with the type of scoliosis caused by neuromuscular disease. This brace is one of a number of devices (thoraco-lumbar-sacral orthoses, or TLSOs) designed to prevent progressive spinal deformity.

The body shell is made of plastic or acrylic materials and may be padded on the inside. The one shown here has two pieces—a front and back shell—which fasten at the sides with Velcro. Many body shells are one-piece devices which open in the front or back and extend over a greater area of the chest. Either type can be worn with other braces and may be used during the day or night or both.

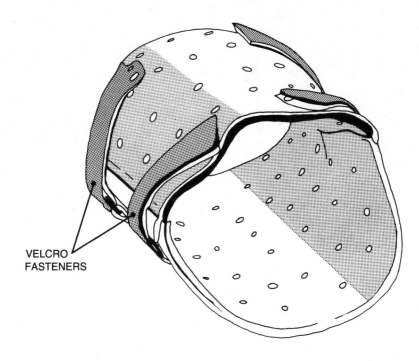

VELCRO
FASTENERS

Body Shell

THE POPE NIGHT SPLINT

Pope night splints help prevent heelcord tightness and joint contractures, which may be caused by muscle imbalance from spasticity or weakness. They are generally worn at night and during naps and are set at 90° (other angles are sometimes recommended).

CALF CUFF

SINGLE UPRIGHT

SHOE

SOLE PLATE

Pope Night Splint

THE LORENZ NIGHT SPLINT (ABDUCTION SPLINT)

This device separates the legs to stretch the adductors, the muscles which bring the legs together. It is usually worn at night and during naps to prevent hip dislocations or partial dislocations (subluxations) in children at risk for malalignments of the hip joints or in children who have had hip surgery. Thigh and pelvic bands are connected by a metal bar that is flared to separate, and sometimes flex, the legs, bringing the thigh bone (femur) and the hip socket (acetabulum) into proper alignment. As with most night braces, the Lorenz night splint may be worn for several months or all through the growing years.

Lorenz Night Splint

THE VARIABLE ABDUCTION HKAFO

The variable abduction HKAFO, developed at the University of Rochester, has a specially designed hip joint which can be adjusted to keep the legs apart, together, or at any desired angle between the two extemes. When set to keep the legs apart, this brace (like the Lorenz night splint) promotes good hip alignment. When set to keep the legs together, it can be used as a frame for standing with assistance, but not for walking. Extensions below the knee help maintain full knee extension and neutral foot alignment. The variable abduction HKAFO is often used for several hours at a time—usually at night. It is appropriate mostly for younger children with myelomeningocele.

HIP AND BACK SUPPORT
WITH SHEEPSKIN LINING

THIGH CUFFS

CALF CUFFS

Variable Abduction HKAFO

THE DENIS-BROWNE SPLINT

The Denis-Browne splint (bar) is commonly applied following serial casting in the treatment of clubfoot. It has also been used to treat twisting (torsion) of bones in the legs or feet, although the benefits of such treatment have not been documented. The length of the bar separating the legs can vary, as can the inward or outward direction of the shoe attachment. Special shoes are attached if necessary.

Denis-Browne Splint

SPECIAL SHOE COMPONENTS

Shoes, which ordinarily provide protection from the elements and irregular ground surfaces, are sometimes modified in an attempt to restore foot balance during standing or walking. Special shoe components or inserts are used by some therapists to improve posture or function or to halt the progression of foot problems. The benefits of special shoes or shoe inserts for the child with a disability have not, however, been confirmed.

Shoes may be specially designed, or regular shoes may be altered, either internally or externally. Common modifications in children's shoes include the addition of components which provide arch support or lateral weight shift. Three such modifications are the Thomas heel, the medial wedge, and the cookie insert.

The Thomas heel

The Thomas heel is an external modification used with children who have foot valgus (falling of the medial foot surface) or outward turning of the feet. The medial extension of the heel provides extra support to the longitudinal arch and helps the foot rotate inward during walking. (A reverse Thomas heel has an extension on the *lateral* heel surface. It is used for foot varus—falling of the lateral foot surface—or for inward turning of the foot.)

THOMAS HEEL

Thomas Heel

The medial wedge

The medial wedge is an external addition to the heel, sole, or both to provide lateral weight shift for treatment of foot valgus. *Lateral* wedges shift weight medially for treatment of foot varus.

MEDIAL WEDGE

Medial Wedge

Cookie insert (arch insole or scaphoid pad)

This internal modification, made of leather or firm sponge material, is placed in the shoe under the inside arch borders to provide support for the longitudinal arch.

COOKIE INSERT

Cookie Insert

INHIBITIVE CASTING

Inhibitive casting has been used by some physical therapists as an adjunct to dynamic treatment: the cast keeps the foot in normal alignment and inhibits unwanted reflexes or muscle tone, allowing the therapist to focus on developing normal movement patterns throughout the rest of the body.

Inhibitive Casting

IMPLICATIONS FOR EDUCATION

The use of braces, shoes, or casts is only one facet of a therapeutic program for abnormalities in muscles and joints. It is generally accompanied by regular range-of-motion exercises and other physical therapy treatments.

Systematic training in ambulation and in performing functional skills—applying and removing ("donning" and "doffing") the brace, rolling over, and attaining a standing position—is best done by a qualified physical therapist. Educators may be asked to ensure that new skills are put into practice in the classroom.

While a brace can be a valuable assistive device for young children, caution is necessary to prevent problems. For instance, metal components of braces should not remain in contact with the skin. Also, because a new brace can cause redness or irritation, it should be applied for gradually increasing time periods until the child develops brace tolerance—a process which may take weeks. This is especially important if the child has a sensory deficit. The child's skin should be inspected for reddened, irritated, or ulcerated areas, and any skin problems should be reported immediately. Braces should be checked for correct fit every four to six months, depending on the child's growth rate, by an orthopedic doctor or a physical therapist.

Cerebral Palsy

Alfred Healy, M.D.

DESCRIPTION

Cerebral palsy (CP), sometimes called chronic, nonprogressive neurologic injury, is a disorder of muscle control or coordination resulting from injury to the brain during its early (fetal, perinatal, and early childhood) stages of development. There may be associated problems with intellectual, visual, or other functions.

With cerebral palsy, the problem lies in the brain's inability to control the muscles; the muscles themselves and the nerves connecting them to the spinal cord are perfectly normal. The extent and location of brain injury determine the type and distribution of CP:

Spasticity

Stiffness of the muscles (hypertonia) occurs when the injury is on the brain surface (motor cortex) or when it involves those nerves leading from the surface through the substance of the brain (corticospinal, or pyramidal, tract) and into the spinal cord. Spasticity is present in about 60 percent of all cases of cerebral palsy.

Dyskinesia

This type, which accounts for roughly 20 percent of all cases of cerebral palsy, is caused by injury to the basal ganglia area, the brain's motor switchboard. Dyskinesia is a term describing the unwanted, involuntary movements of cerebral palsy. These include slow, writhing movements, particularly of the wrist and fingers (athetosis), which may be accompanied by more abrupt and jerky movements (choreoathetosis). Another form of dyskinesia is comprised of slow, rhythmic movements involving the trunk or an entire extremity (dystonia). All three forms are more prominent with voluntary activity or emotional stress. Dyskinesia is sometimes accompanied by increased muscle tone, or "tension," which also varies with body position and emotional state.

Ataxia

Occurring by itself in about 1 percent of all cerebral palsy, ataxia is characterized by a broad-based, lurching gait with primary balance difficulties. The injury is in the cerebellum.

Mixed

Approximately 30 percent of individuals with cerebral palsy have a combination of spasticity and dyskinesia or ataxia, with one type predominating.

With the spastic type of CP, the following terms are used to denote which parts of the body are affected:
* *Dipelgia*—Involvement of the trunk and all four extremeties—the legs more so than the arms
* *Hemiplegia*—Involvement of one side of the body only
* *Paraplegia*—Involvement of the legs only
* *Quadriplegia*—Involvement of both arms, both legs, the head, and the trunk

There are also cases of *monoplegia*—involvement of one extremity—and *triplegia*—involvement of three extremities; but these are unusual.

Some children with cerebral palsy have severe disabilities; others have barely detectable problems with muscle control. There is no universally used, objective method by which physicians or therapists can adequately categorize patients as having mild, moderate, or severe degrees of motor dysfunction. Such estimates are usually made subjectively.

CAUSE

Cerebral palsy results from brain injury due to such events as a stroke during fetal life, lack of oxygen at birth, and intracranial hemorrhage or meningitis during infancy. In as many as 50 percent of the cases, the specific cause of the injury is not evident.

The type of CP is related to three factors: the causal event, the timing of this event, and the location of the damage. For example, an intracranial hemorrhage in a susceptible premature infant may damage the corticospinal and associated tracts, causing spasticity. Or high levels of bilirubin—a product of the breakdown of red blood cells—may damage the basal ganglia in newborns, resulting in athetosis.

INCIDENCE

The incidence of cerebral palsy varies with different studies. The most often quoted figure is 1.5 to 2 per thousand live births. The incidence is higher in areas where there is inadequate prenatal care and accompanying prematurity.

DETECTION

The diagnosis of cerebral palsy is made on the basis of a history of delayed achievement of motor milestones, observation of abnormal movement, and abnormal findings in the physical examination (e.g., stiffness, very active knee jerks, persistent primitive reflexes).

Spasticity or dyskinesia are not always evident during the first few months of life. However, most cases of cerebral palsy can be detected by 12 months, nearly all by 18 months. Some children with abnormalities of posture and movement in the early months reportedly outgrow them; but this, except in mild cases, is rare.

Other factors besides insufficient age can make the diagnosis difficult. These include:

Prematurity

An infant born too early or too small must be given extra time to achieve certain skills. For example, the infant born two months early may be normal but just not sitting up within the normal range of expected times for full-term infants.

Extremes of normal range

Some babies sit at four months, others not until nine months; yet both groups may fall within the normal range. Only when the skill is not being performed after the outer limit of "normal" is reached or when there is a constellation of abnormal signs can we infer that something is wrong.

Quality of performance

Some infants have the ability to manipulate objects at the expected age, yet the manner in which they do so many indicate an abnormality. That is why experienced examiners must observe *how* as well as *when* infants perform motor activities. Since the diagnosis of cerebral palsy is based on clinical judgment and not on blood tests, X-rays, or the like, the observations of skilled examiners are necessary to make or confirm the diagnosis during infancy.

Effects of motor impairment

Children with cerebral palsy, like infants with general developmental delay, often do not perform expected motor tasks at age-appropriate times. It is critically important, however, to differentiate between these two groups of children. The basic indicator is that the generally developmentally delayed child's abilities are depressed in all areas, whereas the child with cerebral palsy may be very depressed in motor activities yet have good socialization and receptive language skills.

The belief that "they will grow out of it"

At times, parents are falsely reassured that, given time, an infant's motor delays will resolve on their own. Also, the physician may be reluctant to make a firm diagnosis of cerebral palsy on the basis of one office visit, particularly if the child is very young. If there is doubt, the wisest course is to reexamine the child at frequent intervals or to make a referral to persons highly experienced in developmental and neurological assessment. The advantages of early treatment if the child does have cerebral palsy—or the relief and reassurance if the child does not—are well worth the extra effort.

COURSE

During infancy, the manifestations of brain injury often change. The initially floppy (hypotonic) baby, for example, can later show signs of spasticity. Sometimes athetosis is not evident until the child is older. For this reason, diagnosis may not be exact in early infancy but may be revised as the child's neuromotor status evolves.

Cerebral palsy is the result of a permanent brain injury and is therefore lifelong. While the brain damage itself is nonprogressive, the resultant muscle control problems are not. However, their progress can be halted— or at least postponed—with proper therapy, including frequent elongation of stiff muscles and proper positioning. In some cases, surgery is necessary to release tight muscles and tendons, particularly of the ankles and hips, or to treat dislocations of the hips. Other orthopedic disorders, such as scoliosis and contractures of the joints, may become more problematic as the child gets older.

When appropriate therapy is available during the child's developing years, the parents can expect to see continued gains in muscle control, strength, and awareness of how certain motor skills are performed; such gains will result in improved ability to move, feed, dress, toilet, or communicate. The rate of this improvement, however, is greatly dependent upon the type of cerebral palsy, the way it is distributed, the degree of muscle involvement, and the presence of associated problems.

Children with cerebral palsy—provided they have comprehensive evaluation, care, and treatment—can look forward to an average longevity. All previous data supporting a shortened life span have been faulted by the inclusion of large numbers of individuals who, at an early age, were placed in institutions where they received less-than-adequate care.

ACCOMPANYING HEALTH PROBLEMS

Events causing brain injury around the time of birth are seldom so site-specific that they bring about only one kind of clinical problem. There are often injuries to different areas of the brain, each of which controls different functions. Associated problems include:

Mental retardation

Around 60 to 70 percent of all children with cerebral palsy are mentally retarded. This problem is seen less often with spastic diplegia.

Visual impairments

As many as 50 percent of all children with spastic cerebral palsy have an eye muscle imbalance problem; refractive errors are almost as common.

Hearing impairment

Cerebral palsy, particularly the type associated with brain damage due to excess bilirubin, may produce hearing deficits (hearing ability should therefore be carefully monitored). Also, children with motor problems may spend a large percentage of their time in a recumbent position; this makes them more susceptible to middle ear infections and persistent fluid in the middle ear, which can cause a conductive hearing loss.

Seizures

The brain injury which results in cerebral palsy often causes scarring on the cortex, a source of chronic irritation that may precipitate seizure activity in 35 to 45 percent (some studies report 60 percent) of persons with cerebral palsy. All types of seizures are reported, grand mal the most frequently.

MEDICAL MANAGEMENT

The interdisciplinary approach

Because the problems associated with cerebral palsy are numerous and complex, treatment involves the integrated efforts of specialists from many disciplines.

The physical therapist works to facilitate motor development, to prevent or slow orthopedic problems (such as limited range of motion or dislocation of joints), and to improve posture and positioning so that the child may more profitably engage in other types of intervention activities.

The occupational therapist teaches parents to handle the child's daily living activities—such as toileting, feeding, and dressing. (In many situations, this service is provided by or shared with the physical therapist.)

Both the physical and occupational therapists may help select appropriate equipment, such as special chairs and eating utensils, to facilitate independence and learning.

The speech pathologist monitors the child's progress in speech and language skills. While it is unlikely that speech therapy *per se* will be initiated before age three, this specialist counsels parents and other therapists on how to stimulate language development and may also work with the occupational therapist in managing feeding problems.

Also important is the primary physician, who treats the usual childhood disorders and helps prevent many health problems from occurring. Depending on the nature of the associated problems, a variety of physician subspecialists may also be involved with the child—an orthopedist to prescribe braces or perform surgical procedures, an ophthalmologist to treat crossed eyes (strabismus), a neurologist to help control seizures.

Muscle relaxants

Certain drugs are helpful in cases of hypertonia. The three most commonly used are diazepam, dantrolene, and baclofen. Diazepam (Valium) acts on the central nervous system rather than directly on the muscle. This drug is useful for treating spinal cord injury as well as cerebral palsy. Diazepam may cause physical dependency and therefore should not be withdrawn suddenly.

Dantrolene (Dantrium) works directly on the muscle, reducing contraction. It is especially useful with children whose care is made difficult by prolonged muscle contraction and who will not be troubled by a reduction in voluntary muscle power. This drug may affect liver function; therefore, signs of jaundice should be reported immediately.

Baclofen (Lioresal) acts mainly on the spinal cord to relieve increased muscle tone and muscle spasms. It is used primarily with spinal cord lesions and occasionally for cerebral palsy. The most common side effect is sedation, which tends to disappear a few days after the initial doses.

IMPLICATIONS FOR EDUCATION

Some children with cerebral palsy have normal intelligence, which is masked by severe motor impairment. (With motorically handicapped individuals, accurate assessment of cognitive abilities can be difficult.) Most, however, have some degree of cognitive delay. Both groups require a program and environment that is optimal for learning. When devising a home- or center-based learning program, educators need to consider the limitations brought about by the child's motor and possible cognitive deficits; unrealistic expectations can be frustrating to both child and parents. Educators need to be especially patient with these children; studies show that they require a longer than usual period to respond to a request.

Most children with CP should avoid constant sitting, especially "W" sitting; instead they should assume different positions in order to prevent further tightening of muscles. Too, they need proper equipment to facilitate eye-hand coordination, necessary for learning and for the performance of self-help skills.

Educators, who have regular contact with the child and family, can reinforce the advice of therapists and other service providers.

SEE ALSO

Bracing, Neuroanatomy, The Neurological Examination, Orthopedic Problems, Perinatal Injury, Positioning, and *Seizure Disorders*

Child Abuse and Neglect

Gerald Solomons, M.D.

DEFINITION

The definition of child maltreatment is a legal one and varies from state to state. It can include physical or emotional abuse or neglect and sexual abuse. A broad definition is found in the **Child Abuse Prevention and Treatment Act,** Public Law 93-247: "The physical or mental injury, sexual abuse or exploitation, negligent treatment or maltreatment of a child under the age of eighteen . . . by a person who is responsible for the child's welfare . . .."

INCIDENCE

The actual incidence of child abuse and neglect is unknown. The commonly accepted figure is one million cases per year, but some investigators believe that if all forms of abuse are included in the definition this figure would be as high as four to five million. About five thousand children die from child abuse each year. Approximately one-third of the incidents of physical abuse occur in children under five. Sexual abuse is three to four times more common than physical abuse; neglect is five to eight times more common.

Child abuse occurs at all socioeconomic and educational levels, though it is more often reported among lower socioeconomic groups. Parents are not the only abusers; others include stepparents, boyfriends, babysitters, and foster parents. Around 60 to 90 percent of abusers have been victims themselves. Less than 10 percent are severely emotionally disturbed.

ABUSE AND NEGLECT OF THE CHILD WITH DIS-ABILITIES

Child abuse is more likely to occur when (1) there is stress and strain in the family; (2) parents have unrealistic expectations of the child; or (3) parents are emotionally and socially isolated. Usually, one particular child in the family serves as scapegoat, receiving the brunt of the abuser's animosity. Low-birth-weight infants, while they comprise only 10 percent of newborns, make up approximately 20 to 25 percent of the physically abused population. A major factor here may be impairment of maternal-infant attachment.

Children with disabilities are also particularly vulnerable. The mere physical care of a disabled child can be exceedingly taxing—physically, emotionally, and financially. When these stresses are compounded by parental anger, denial, and guilt—and by long periods without child-care relief—the potential for abuse increases dramatically.

Approximately one-third of abused children have signs of central nervous system damage, one-half to two-thirds have intellectual impairment, and one-third are below the normal range for height and weight. While many children are already disabled prior to being abused, the abuse itself frequently results in developmental disabilities, including neurological impairment. The effects of neglect can be just as devastating as those of physical abuse.

All maltreated children have serious long-term psychosocial problems. In a recent study in a cerebral palsy clinic, issues of child abuse were important considerations in deciding on the custody of 36 out of 86 children. Nearly one-half of this group (17 of 36) were injured severely enough by abusers in the home to warrant custody by the state.

There is significant potential for abuse by those caring for handicapped children, including medical and education-related professionals. The professional also wields tremendous power over children with handicaps and their families by determining the type, nature, and extent of services received and even whether some children will be excluded from services. When trying to develop the maximum potential of the handicapped child, care should be taken not to trigger abuse and neglect by raising unrealistic expectations for performance or by otherwise altering a climate of acceptance in the family.

SIGNS OF CHILD ABUSE

Because the definition of child abuse varies from state to state, it is difficult to name specific indications. They include burns, bruises, abrasions—anything that could result from an ordinary accident. Many signs in the child's appearance and behavior and in the behavior of the parent or caretaker may arouse suspicion. One sign alone may mean nothing or have a reasonable explanation. If there are a number of signs, however, or if they occur frequently, there is cause for suspicion. A major indication is a discrepancy between the injury itself and the story of how it happened.

REPORTING CHILD ABUSE

Every state has a law requiring health and other professionals to report child abuse whenever it is suspected. In many states there are penalties for professionals who fail to report. These include a jail sentence and/or a fine of several hundred dollars; in some cases the professional who fails to report child abuse can be liable for damages resulting from subsequent injury to the child.

Know your state law in detail, particularly the definition of child abuse and neglect; know also the reporting procedure if you are a mandatory reporter and the legal consequences if you do not report. Utilize the child abuse law as a means of getting help early to a family in need. And, most importantly, be compassionate, sympathetic and understanding. Under certain circumstances, many of us could become child abusers.

Cleft Lip and Palate

James C. Hardy, Ph.D.

DESCRIPTION

During the sixth through the thirteenth weeks of fetal life, the roof and upper front of the mouth are formed by development and fusion, mostly in the midline, of soft tissue and bony processes. Interruption of this formation results in a group of disorders known as clefts.

(1) The central portion of the **UPPER LIP**

(2) and the **PREMAXILLA** evolve from the nasal structures. They fuse with the lateral lip tissues and upper jaw bones to form the upper lip and jaw.

(3) This fusion completes the **ALVEOLAR PROCESS**—the gum ridge from which the teeth will erupt.

(4) The bones of the hard palate, or **PALATAL PROCESS OF THE MAXILLARY BONES AND PALATAL BONES,** begin to develop to the midline and, from front to back, fuse with each other and with the bony partition (nasal septum, not shown) which separates the two nostrils.

(5) Lastly the tissues of the soft palate, or **VELUM PALATUM,** evolve and fuse in the midline.

(6) These tissues and those of the **PHARYNGEAL WALLS**

(7) form the **VELOPHARYNGEAL PORT,** surrounded by a muscular sphincter that normally closes during eating, drinking, and swallowing.

Fusion of premaxilla and maxillary bones

Fusion of palatal processes of maxilla

Fusion of palatal bones

Normal Development of the Lip and Palate

The specific forms and severity of clefts vary, and these variations are usually attributed to the timing of the interference with normal development.

Cleft of the lip only

Interference during the initial stages of development is likely to result in a cleft of the lip only. This malformation may include as little as the border of the lip or it may extend upward and into the nostril (as shown).

Cleft of the Lip Only

Clefts of the lip and palate

Clefts of both the lip and palate appear to result from an impediment to normal development that spans weeks six through thirteen of fetal life.

Unilateral Cleft of the Lip and Palate — *The premaxilla and the maxilla fuse on one side only, as do the bones of the hard palate and the nasal septum. There is a cleft of the tissues of the soft palate.*

Bilateral Cleft of the Lip and Palate — *Neither side of the premaxilla, the maxilla, or the palatal bones fuse together.*

Clefts of the palate only

Interference during the later stages of development may result in clefts of palatal tissues only.

Cleft of the Soft Palate Only

Cleft of Both the Hard and Soft Palates

Normal development of the lip and the hard and soft palates is essential to proper eating and speech production. The front lip helps control liquids and foods during drinking and eating and helps create a suction to assist in moving liquids and foods to the back of the mouth for swallowing. The hard palate provides a partition between the mouth and nasal passages. The muscles of the soft palate normally act in conjunction with those of the walls of the upper throat (pharyngeal walls) to close the opening between the posterior oral and nasal cavities (velopharyngeal port) during eating, drinking, and swallowing.

An opening between the nasal and oral cavities has two adverse effects upon speech production. First, the quality of speech is likely to be offensive; the voice has a "nasal" quality when the air in the nasal cavity is set into vibration along with the air in the throat and oral cavity. Second and most importantly, the buildup of air pressure within the oral cavity that is necessary to produce many consonant sounds is negated by the leak through the nasal cavity. In addition to causing speech impediments, an opening between the oral and nasal cavities leads to increased susceptibility to upper respiratory infections.

Clefts also affect hearing. Normal hearing is dependent upon proper functioning of the eustachian tubes, which provide an opening between the middle ear and the posterior nasal cavity. With a cleft palate, the eustachian tube is exposed to foods and liquids, predisposing it to inflammation. Also, the frequent upper respiratory infections common in children with clefts increase the likelihood of eustachian tube and middle ear infections.

The congenital anomaly of clefting, then, may result in the following problems, the presence or severity of which depends on the specific characteristics of the cleft and the particular child:

- Serious dental problems, including inappropriate alignment of the teeth and/or a faulty relationship between the upper and lower teeth (malocclusion)
- Susceptibility to upper respiratory infections
- Middle ear disease and associated hearing impairment from eustachian tube dysfunction
- Significant feeding difficulties and subsequent nutritional problems in early life
- Problems of speech development
- Psychosocial problems and low self-esteem due to **(1)** strained parent-child relationships, **(2)** facial disfigurement, **(3)** a speech problem, and/or **(4)** a hearing impairment
- Educational difficulties due to health, hearing, and psychosocial problems

Babies with clefts may have additional congenital anomalies, such as heart defects and extra fingers or toes.

CAUSE

There is no comprehensive, definitive explanation for cleft lip or palate. Certain families may have a history of clefts, especially clefts of the palate only. Even for that subgroup, however, the exact pattern of genetic transmission is not usually clear. A number of environmental factors are also believed to result in clefting, including German measles, drugs, and vitamin deficiencies in the mother. Any genetic pattern for, or predisposition to, clefts is compounded by the possible presence of these factors.

INCIDENCE

Known racial differences make general overall incidence figures meaningless. For example, with Caucasians, cleft lip and/or palate occurs in one of every 550 live births; with Blacks, it occurs in only one of every 2,500 live births.

DETECTION

A cleft can usually be detected at birth. Exceptions are submucous clefts of the palate, in which the posterior portion of the palatal bones are not fused. With this condition, the tissue of the soft palate may appear normal anatomically, and the cleft may not become evident until a feeding and/or speech development problem appears.

COURSE AND INTERDISCIPLINARY MANAGEMENT

Proper management of cleft problems requires highly specialized interdisciplinary efforts.

Cleft treatment centers

Infants with clefts should be referred to one of the numerous cleft treatment centers that have been established throughout the nation. (Locations of interdisciplinary cleft lip and palate treatment centers may be obtained by contacting the American Cleft Palate Educational Foundation, 331 Salk Hall, University of Pittsburgh, Pittsburgh, PA 15261.)

The staffs of cleft treatment centers usually provide a variety of services:
- Surgeons repair the cleft.
- Otolaryngologists diagnose and treat ear disease and eustachian tube dysfunction.
- Pediatricians diagnose any additional birth defects, evaluate general health status, and provide general medical treatment.
- Orthodontists anticipate and work to prevent problems of dental occlusion.
- Prosthodontists construct any needed intra-oral appliances to provide missing teeth and/or a partition between the oral and nasal cavities.
- Pedodontists oversee dental development and hygiene.

- Speech-language pathologists advise and plan programs relative to speech development.
- Audiologists assist the otolaryngologist in determining the presence and type of hearing impairment and recommend hearing aids when appropriate.

In addition to these specialists, treatment centers often have sophisticated radiology services which provide documentation of the effects of growth as well as surgical and dental procedures. They may also have psychologists, social service workers, and appropriately trained nurses to assist parents and other family members with potential problems.

Management

Though it is desirable to surgically close clefts as soon as possible, surgery during the first or second month of life may interfere with the growth of the maxillofacial structures. Surgical closure of clefts of the lip may be done when the infant is three to six months old. Initial surgery of the palate may be delayed until the child is twelve to eighteen months old. The final surgeries to bring about optimum cosmetic results may not be performed until adolesence to allow for final growth.

In general, the management goals for clefts of the lip and palate, and for clefts of the palate only, are to make the oral cavity structurally sufficient to reduce both feeding difficulties and hearing problems by the time the child is three to four years old. For a great number of cases, however, achieving adequate palatal function (velopharyngeal competence) for speech production must await secondary surgical procedures and/or prosthetic management during the early school years.

During the formative period of speech development, the child who is unable to produce a number of speech sounds due to a cleft of the palate may learn inappropriate compensatory speech production patterns. While those components of speech that are deviant due to mislearning may change as a result of management by a speech-language pathologist, the child still may not be able to completely eliminate the speech production problems until the cleft treatment team is able to restore adequate palatal functioning.

IMPLICATIONS FOR EDUCATION

The cleft palate team will make recommendations for specific management techniques, since these vary with the individual. Feeding techniques, for example, will be quite different for a cleft of the lip than for a cleft of the palate. With the former, the infant cannot close the mouth around the nipple to create suction; with the latter, liquids are forced into the nasal cavity, sometimes to the extent of being expelled from the nostrils.

The child may have to be kept on soft foods for an extended period because of problems with development of teeth.

Because of increased susceptibility, unnecessary exposure to upper respiratory infections should be avoided. However, precautions should not extend to excluding the child from early educational experiences which may be beneficial. Certain modifications in the environment (e.g., increased humidity in the classroom) may help reduce the extent and severity of these infections.

In cases where there is hearing loss, educational methods appropriate for the hearing impaired should be employed.

Parents of children with clefts need to have professionals with whom they can discuss their ongoing concerns about health, growth, and development; they also need continuing support to offset guilt reactions and other negative feelings.

SEE ALSO
Middle Ear Disease

The Colostomy and Ileostomy

Marcia Henderson, R.N., M.A., C.P.N.P.
Janet R. Mapel, R.N., B.S.N., C.P.N.P.

DESCRIPTION

Both a colostomy and an ileostomy involve the construction of an artificial opening, called a stoma, into the intestine through the abdominal wall. The bowel contents are diverted through the stoma, which may be temporary or permanent, into a collection appliance. This is usually a disposable plastic bag which is held in place over the stoma by self-sticking adhesive and/or a belt. The remaining section of the bowel may or may not be present.

There are four major types of intestinal stomas, two of which will be discussed in detail in this chapter.

Colostomy

A colostomy is a diversion of the large intestine, or colon.

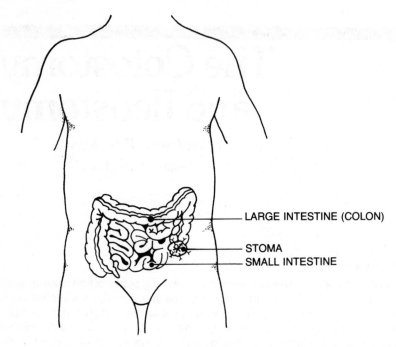

LARGE INTESTINE (COLON)

STOMA
SMALL INTESTINE

Site of Stoma for a Colostomy

The contents of the lower (sigmoid) colon—solid or semi-solid stool—are generally not irritating to the skin. An appliance is therefore not always necessary, though one may be used nonetheless for ease of collection.

Ileostomy

This is a diversion of the lower third of the small intestine, known as the ileum. The intestinal contents of the ileum are liquid and highly erosive to the skin, requiring both meticulous protection from stoma discharge and the wearing of an appliance.

Urinary conduit

Urine is directed from the kidneys and ureters through the stoma via a passageway constructed from a portion of the small intestine (ileum). The removal of the portion of small intestine does not affect bowel function; the intestinal contents (stool) continue to pass through the rectum.

Because urine is highly erosive to the skin, the child must wear an appliance.

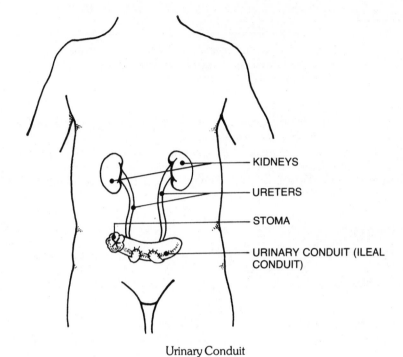

Urinary Conduit

Cutaneous fistula

This is a very small opening from the intestine or urinary tract through the surface of the abdominal wall. It may arise spontaneously or as a result of surgery. The drainage through a cutaneous fistula may be stool, urine, or mucus, any of which is highly erosive to the skin and may require the wearing of an appliance.

CAUSE

In very young children, some of the most common reasons for a colostomy/ileostomy are:
- Congenital absence of the nerve endings that cause feces to be propelled through the colon, rectum, and anus (Hirschsprung disease)
- An anus and/or rectum that is not formed properly so that there is no exit for the feces (anorectal atresia)
- Inflammatory bowel disease (necrotizing enterocolitis of premature infants)

The ostomy is usually a temporary diversion until the primary condition is alleviated, at which time the bowel is reattached and the ostomy closed.

INCIDENCE

Both Hirschsprung disease and congenital anorectal malformations occur in approximately one in five thousand live births. The occurrence of other diseases which necessitate a colostomy or ileostomy varies.

DETECTION

Disorders necessitating an ostomy diversion are usually detected at birth or soon after, though some obstructive bowel diseases (e.g., Hirschsprung disease) may not be diagnosed for a year or two, or even longer. Anorectal anomalies are generally readily visible at birth. Such examinations as a barium enema (X-ray) will help the physician determine what part of the bowel is involved and how serious the obstruction may be.

COURSE

Most colostomies in young children are temporary, lasting a few months to a few years. Once the bowel is reconnected, only a small abdominal scar remains.

ACCOMPANYING HEALTH PROBLEMS

Since the ostomy diverts bowel contents, health problems are usually related to digestion, particularly of foods that cause diarrhea. When there are accompanying nutrient absorption disorders, growth must be closely monitored.

MANAGEMENT

Elimination

Both an ileostomy and a colostomy usually require an appliance to collect the fecal material and protect the skin. The permanent or long-term appliance consists of a collecting bag or pouch, faceplate, and belt (particularly helpful with the ambulatory child). Some bags are disposable and changed daily; others are open at the lower end to allow for regular emptying of the contents. A clamp closure may be used with the child who is old enough not to lie on the clamp and cause trauma to the sensitive stoma. Rubber band closure is a safe alternative for the younger child.

If the child has a temporary colostomy, the lower bowel continues, despite disuse, to secrete mucus. As a result, there may be drainage from the rectum, which diapers or panties are generally sufficient to absorb.

FACEPLATE

BELT

COLLECTING BAG WITH CLAMP

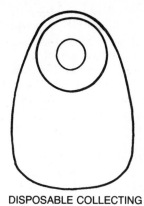

DISPOSABLE COLLECTING BAG

Collection Appliances

STOMA

Faceplate of a Collection Appliance
(Placed Over the Stoma)

Diet and fluid intake

Children with a colostomy or ileostomy need a balanced diet that is sufficient to promote growth. This should include enough fiber/residue for stool formation. It will be evident which foods the child cannot tolerate and should therefore avoid.

Since fluids may be lost quickly due to decreased absorption from the colon, the child needs to drink plenty of liquids. Children with an ileostomy have a precarious fluid and electrolyte balance; a mild diarrhea can progress in only a few hours to a life-threatening situation.

Skin care

Skin care is an ongoing and critical concern while the child has an ostomy. Any itching or burning under the appliance means there is leakage and that the appliance needs to be changed. Children who have no skin sensation may not feel itching or burning. In such cases, the appliance should be inspected three to four times daily—with each toileting or diaper change, perhaps, or following meals.

Odor and/or gas

Some odor and/or gas is fairly common with a colostomy. Certain foods create more gas than others; while these need not be eliminated from the diet, they should be controlled if they cause social embarassment. The new appliances rarely transmit odor from gas or feces unless there is leakage. Some families utilize deodorants specifically designed for these appliances. Regular changing of the appliance with attention to cleaning (e.g., washing the belts) helps control offensive odors.

IMPLICATIONS FOR EDUCATION

The child who is at an appropriate developmental level may be involved in the care of the colostomy by handing articles to the caretaker or by helping to empty the bag. Such involvement may enhance the child's self-esteem and control of body functions. All materials necessary to change the appliance should be at hand. These fit easily into a medium-sized cosmetic bag, which can be carried in a purse or a school bag. Keeping the specific supplies at hand encourages routine changing, which helps to prevent skin irritation and soiled clothing. The parent or primary caretaker is a good source of information regarding appropriate methods for removing and applying the appliance.

The colostomy and ileostomy present no physical limitations. The child may lie on his stomach and may be held and handled the same as any other child. Even swimming is permissible. However, nothing should ever be introduced into the stoma.

The following signs and symptoms should be reported to the parent or primary caretaker promptly:
- Excessive bleeding from the stoma
- Copious watery diarrhea
- No passage of gas or fecal material from the stoma
- Pencil-thin feces
- Bloating (abdominal distention), pain, tenderness, fever, vomiting, or increased irritability
- Redness and/or abrasion of the skin surrounding the stoma
- Any unusual out-pouching of the stoma

Computerized Axial Tomography (CAT) and Other Imaging Techniques

Frederick R. Schultz, M.D.

DESCRIPTION

CAT scanning is a radiologic technique which allows for precise examination of internal body structures. With ordinary X-ray, a single beam passes through the body and strikes an X-ray film, producing a photographic negative. In contrast, a CAT scanner passes multiple X-ray beams through the body at different angles, generating, with the use of a computer, a composite image. A series of images is generally made, displaying numerous cross sections ("slices") of any part of the body. This technique makes it possible to focus clearly on structures as small as two millimeters thick.

Cat Scan of a Normal Brain

Cat Scan Showing Dilated Ventricles

When CAT scanning was made available in the early 1970s, its primary application was in identifying abnormalities within the brain and its coverings. Since that time, its use has expanded tremendously; today CAT scanning permits close analysis of virtually any structure of the body.

A child or infant must remain perfectly still during the scanning procedure. Initially, this took up to 20 minutes, and children had to be sedated with medication; some even required a general anesthetic. CAT scanners now operate much more rapidly—about three seconds per slice. However, sedation with medication (with possible, though rare, complications or side effects) is still necessary with children who are likely to move. Depending on the degree of sedation required and the period of time necessary for it to wear off, these children may need to remain at the scanning facility for up to several hours. At times, particularly with small infants, hospital admission may be advisable.

Cat Scanner

CAT scanning, like an ordinary X-ray, is painless. While the amount of radiation associated with this technique exceeds that of an ordinary X-ray, the small amount of tissue exposed keeps the dosage within an acceptable range.

USES

The primary use of CAT scanning with children has been for quick identification of abnormalities in the brain and its coverings, including tumors, bleeding, infection, hydrocephalus, or various congenital anomalies.

CAT scanning has to a large extent replaced other, more complicated radiographic procedures, such as pneumoencephalography (which involves injecting air into the spaces within the brain) and cerebral angiography (which involves injecting X-ray contrast materials into blood vessels going to the brain).

BENEFITS

Besides being rapid and accurate, CAT scanning imparts much more information than is attainable from ordinary X-rays. Too, the results are available immediately. CAT scanning is not painful and carries considerably less risk of complication than do procedures such as pneumoencephalography or cerebral angiography.

OTHER IMAGING TECHNIQUES

Positron emission tomography (PET)

Like CAT scanning, PET scanning visualizes brain "slices." However, this technique has an added advantage: it measures the metabolism of each small area of the brain. With PET scanning, physicians may be able to determine which parts of the brain are affected during various disease states, thereby learning more about such conditions as epilepsy, metabolic diseases, and certain psychiatric disorders.

Nuclear magnetic resonance (NMR)

This technique is based on the tendency of hydrogen ions in body tissues to "line up" when placed in a strong magnetic field. When lined up, the ions react in a predictable manner to various radio frequencies. This produces a "map" of hydrogen ion densities, which, when processed by a computer, creates pictures of the scanned portion of the body. A major advantage of NMR scanning is that there is no radiation exposure. Also, the same equipment can create several different diagnostically useful images simultaneously.

Ultrasonography

Ultrasonic waves, sound waves which vibrate at such high frequencies that they are not audible to the human ear, are bounced off body tissues (a particular organ, a tumor, a developing fetus). Their "echoes" are transmitted electronically to a screen, creating a realistic image which can be photographed or viewed directly. This technique is used for determining gestational age, for prenatal diagnosis of birth defects, and for detecting bleeding into the brain and resultant hydrocephalus in premature infants. There is no radiation (X-ray) exposure with ultrasound. Used appropriately, it is considered to be quite safe.

Congenital Heart Disease

James A. Blackman, M.D.

DESCRIPTION

Congenital heart disease (CHD) includes cardiovascular malformations which are present and usually evident at the time of birth, but which may not be recognized until months or even years later.

The body is dependent upon the heart to pump oxygen and nutrients to all its tissues; therefore, physiologic, anatomic, or electrical defects are debilitating and potentially life-threatening. The more common heart defects include coarctation of the aorta, patent ductus arteriosus (PDA), atrial septal defect (ASD), ventricular septal defect (VSD), tetralogy of Fallot (TOF), and transposition of the great arteries (TGA):

Coarctation of the aorta

A narrowing of the aorta causes the left ventricle to pump harder, raising the blood pressure above the constricted part and lowering it in the blood vessels below.

Patent ductus arteriosus

The duct used to bypass the lungs in the fetus remains open after birth. Oxygenated blood from the left side of the heart flows across the duct, back into the pulmonary artery; this makes the left ventricle work harder and floods the lungs.

Atrial septal defect

Blood leaks through a hole in the wall from the left to the right side, enlarging the right atrium and ventricle as well as the pulmonary artery.

Ventricular septal defect

Blood leaks through a hole in the wall between the ventricles, usually from left to right. Large defects may strain both ventricles, particularly the left.

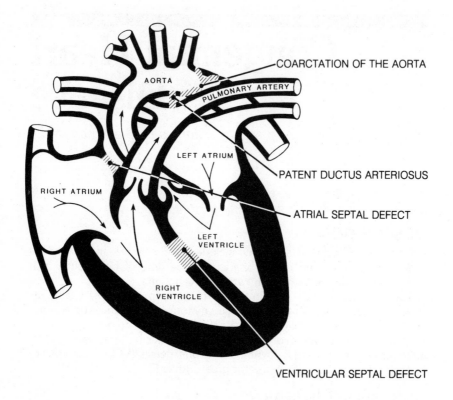

Common Heart Defects

Tetralogy of Fallot

A combination of four defects causes deoxygenated blood to mix with oxygenated blood and be carried to the body:

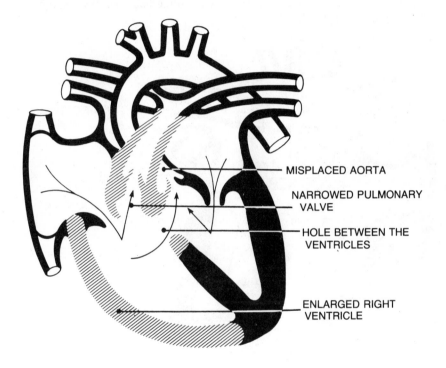

MISPLACED AORTA

NARROWED PULMONARY VALVE

HOLE BETWEEN THE VENTRICLES

ENLARGED RIGHT VENTRICLE

Tetralogy of Fallot

Transposition of the great arteries

The aorta and pulmonary artery are attached to the wrong ventricles. Deoxygenated blood is carried to the body, oxygenated blood to the lungs. A patent ductus arteriosus and septal defect, if present, allow some oxygenated blood to reach the rest of the body, making life possible. Newborns with this defect usually require immediate palliative surgery prior to definitive correction.

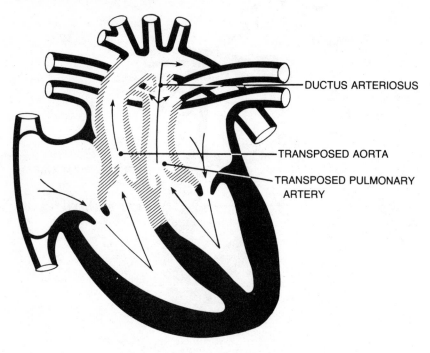

DUCTUS ARTERIOSUS

TRANSPOSED AORTA

TRANSPOSED PULMONARY ARTERY

Transposition of the Great Arteries

CAUSE

When the embryo is just 23 days old, the heart begins to beat. The rapidly developing heart is particularly susceptible to deleterious influences during early fetal life. In most cases the specific cause for congenital heart disease is not identifiable. There is a suspected association with teratogens—that is, agents or factors (viruses, drugs, excessive radiation) which cause physical defects in the developing embryo. However, there are cases of identical twins in which one developed CHD and the other did not, even though both were presumably exposed to the same environment in the uterus. CHD may also be caused by new gene mutations and other genetic factors. (It is linked, for example, with a number of chromosomal abnormalities, including those responsible for Down and Turner syndromes.)

INCIDENCE

About eight out of every thousand people have cardiovascular malformations. The chances of having a second child with a heart defect is 2
to 5 percent; they may be even greater if two children in one family
are already affected. The prevalence of malformations among children
whose parents have congenital heart disease is 3 to 4 percent.

DETECTION

Serious CHD is often recognizable at birth; the newborn shows breathing
difficulties and remains blue despite the administration of high concentrations of oxygen. While the physical examination, chest X-ray, and tracing
of the electrical activity of the heart (electrocardiogram) may indicate the
presence of heart disease, other, more sophisticated tests are often necessary to determine the type. One newer, useful diagnostic technique is
echocardiography: sound waves are bounced off the heart to produce
an image of its structures on paper or a television screen. It is sometimes
necessary to obtain an exact outline of the heart structures and to chart
the flow of blood through it by a procedure called cardiac catheterization,
which involves injecting dye into the heart via a tube threaded through
blood vessels.

COURSE

How seriously the child will be affected by congenital heart disease
depends upon the type and severity of the problem. Some defects (ASD,
VSD) may be so minor that the child will tolerate them well and no
specific corrective procedures will be necessary. In such cases, the child's
condition is followed very closely, and corrective procedures are considered
only if there are signs of worsening. Severe malformations, however, such
as those in which the blood bypasses the lungs (TGA or TOF), can be
life-threatening unless treated early. If, due to small size or poor health,
the child is not able to withstand major corrective surgery, it may be
necessary to perform temporary surgical procedures which allow for adequate oxygenation of the blood.

ACCOMPANYING HEALTH PROBLEMS

During the first few years of life, children with significant heart defects
are often in and out of the hospital, where they are treated not only
for the heart condition but also for secondary medical problems, such
as pneumonias, poor feeding, or infections. Other secondary problems
are of particular importance. Among these is congestive heart failure, a
condition in which the heart, having to work extra hard, becomes strained
and does not pump as efficiently as it should, causing fluid to back up
into the lungs, liver, and other organs. Drugs such as digitalis and water

pills (diuretics) are generally effective in preventing and treating this complication.

The altered anatomy of the heart, including narrowed valves or holes
between heart chambers, is conducive to the growth of bacteria, which
can damage the heart even further. Clumps of bacteria may even break
off and lodge in the brain, causing abscesses. Such serious complications
must be identified and treated with antibiotics as quickly as possible.

The degree of severity of congenital heart disease determines the effects
it will have on growth and development. The incomplete oxygenation
of blood and extra caloric expenditure that accompany the most severe
forms of this condition result in poor growth of tissue, causing the child
to be small and underdeveloped. Serious conditions also cause poor appetite (with resultant inadequate caloric intake) and frequent hospitalizations
for surgery and secondary illnesses. The less severe types of heart defects,
on the other hand, are not likely to significantly interfere with normal
growth and development.

MEDICAL MANAGEMENT

The main features of management include early identification, medical
and physical stabilization prior to corrective surgery, rehabilitation following
surgery, and—of special importance—nutritional and developmental assessment and treatment before, during, and after surgery.

IMPLICATIONS FOR EDUCATION

Oftentimes, frequent hospitalization, coupled with the unstable medical
condition of children with congenital heart disease, diverts attention away
from learning and development. It is almost impossible to determine the
potential for children in such circumstances. Nevertheless, growth of the
brain and other tissues is rapid during the first several years, and attention
to developmental needs cannot be postponed until after surgery and medical management are complete. Thus, early intervention professionals in
home- or center-based programs must work closely with the medical team
to determine how the child's development can be coordinated most efficiently with medical management. Once early intervention personnel understand both the nature of the heart condition and the rationale for
treatment, they can bring their performance expectations in line with the
child's physical limitations. They can also observe the child for fatigue,
poor appetite, or other warning signs of setbacks or complications. Congenital heart disease is a good example of how important it is for medical
and education-related professionals to work together for the child's optimal
treatment in the early years.

SEE ALSO

Low Birth Weight and *Teratogens*

Congenital Infections

James A. Blackman, M.D.

Congenital infections comprise a group of diseases acquired either before or during birth through exposure to viral, bacterial, or protozoan organisms. Besides causing illness and death in the newborn period, they may result in chronic physical, sensory, and mental handicaps. Although many infections may cause damage to the fetus and newborn, this chapter is limited to the so-called STORCH diseases, which are particularly significant in causing developmental disabilities.

Syphilis

Toxoplasmosis

Other infections

Rubella

Cytomegalic inclusion disease

Herpes

SYPHILIS

Syphilis is a sexually transmitted infection caused by the bacterium *Treponema pallidum*. Untreated syphilis in the mother, whether contracted during pregnancy or years before, may be transmitted to the fetus. In 25 percent of cases, untreated syphilis in a pregnant woman results in the death of the fetus, usually during the second trimester. An additional 25 percent die soon after birth. Of those who live, about 25 percent show signs of jaundice, anemia, pneumonia, skin rash, and bone inflammation. The remaining 75 percent may show no signs of infection at birth yet later manifest such problems as abnormalities of the teeth, blindness, skeletal anomalies, mental retardation, and sensorineural deafness.

The exact incidence of congenital syphilis is dependent upon the incidence of untreated syphilis in pregnant women. With the advent of effective antibiotics, this figure has been decreasing. Since early treatment may help prevent defects, it is important that all pregnant women have a blood test for syphilis in the early stages of pregnancy. Once the mother has been adequately treated, there is no risk in future pregnancies (unless she becomes reinfected with syphilis).

Whenever a newborn has general signs of infection, the possibility of syphilis in the mother should be investigated. The diagnosis of congenital syphilis is confirmed by a special blood test (called VDRL or FTA) or, less commonly, by viewing the organism under a microscope. If the results suggest congenital syphilis, treatment with appropriate antibiotics, usually penicillin, should begin immediately. These infants must be followed closely for at least 12 months to insure that the treatment is effective. More specific medical management is dependent upon the organ systems affected.

Because children with congenital syphilis may require special education for their sensory or mental handicaps, it is important for educators to understand which organ systems are primarily affected. If the infant has been appropriately treated, there is no risk of infection to those caring for the child.

TOXOPLASMOSIS

Toxoplasmosis is an infection caused by the protozoan organism *Toxoplasma gondii*. Although this organism infects many animals, including humans, the cat is the most widely recognized vector of transmission. Cysts containing the organism are passed through the animal's feces to the soil, which becomes potentially infective. Toxoplasmosis can also be contracted by ingesting the raw meat or eggs of infected animals. Since an infected individual is usually without symptoms, the organism may pass through the placenta of an unsuspecting pregnant woman and into the fetus.

Toxoplasmosis may result in spontaneous abortion or premature delivery. Affected infants are characterized by low birth weight, a large liver and spleen, jaundice, and anemia. Congenital defects include hydrocephalus, microcephaly, and calcifications in the brain. Some of the problems which may become manifest later are mental retardation, seizures, cerebral palsy, and disease of the retina with resultant blindness.

The approximate incidence of congenital toxoplasmosis is about one to two per thousand live births. This condition should be suspected in any infant who shows signs of congenital infection. Diagnosis is confirmed by a specific blood test or, rarely, by isolating the organism from body tissues. Antiprotozoan drugs, although their efficacy has yet to be scientifically proven, are used to treat the disease in the newborn period in hopes of preventing further damage by the organism.

Because toxoplasmosis is normally not transmitted from person to person, individuals caring for affected infants are not in danger of catching it. Once the mother is treated, there is no danger to the fetus during a future pregnancy.

The severity of this disease calls for individualized educational programs involving many professionals.

OTHER INFECTIONS

Other infectious agents, including influenza virus, chicken pox, and various enteroviruses (such as Coxsackie and ECHO), are suspected of causing damage to the fetus; but since their effects are still uncertain, they will not be discussed in this chapter.

RUBELLA

Rubella, commonly called German measles, is a virus which usually produces only mild upper respiratory symptoms and rash in the infected individual. It can, however, cause severe damage to the fetus—in some cases resulting in spontaneous abortion. When women are infected during the first month of pregnancy, there is a 35 percent chance that the fetus will be affected. This figure decreases to 25 percent in the second month, 16 percent in the third. When women are infected after the fourth month of pregnancy, damage to the fetus is uncommon.

Except during epidemics, the incidence of babies affected by rubella in the uterus is estimated at between 0.1 and 0.7 per thousand live births. This represents a drop from previous years, presumably as a result of recent mass immunization for rubella. If the immunization rate decreases, however, or if the immunity achieved from immunization in infancy proves to wear off in adulthood, the incidence figure could rise. While there is no specific treatment for the infection, it can be prevented through effective immunization of everyone.

Rubella in the newborn should be suspected whenever an infant shows the general signs of a congenital infection, particularly if the mother has had flu-like illness during pregnancy; the diagnosis is confirmed by isolating the virus and by blood tests. Affected newborns may also have a low birth weight, a large liver and spleen, and a peculiar rash (petechiae), caused by the leakage of minute amounts of blood into the skin. Typical congenital malformations include heart defects, microcephaly, cataracts, and small eyes (microphthalmia). Later complications may occur in infants who are asymptomatic at birth. Thus, it is possible to trace to congenital infections a hearing loss which manifests itself months or years after birth. Other later complications may include mental retardation, seizures, thyroid disease, and diabetes.

Infected infants may continue to excrete the virus for up to 12 months. Therefore, susceptible personnel who are pregnant should avoid contact with infants with proven rubella. In addition, all women of childbearing age who have contact with young children, particularly with children who have a high prevalence of congenital infections, should have a blood test to determine their immunity to rubella. Susceptible women should avoid contact with such infants or be immunized at a time when there is no risk of pregnancy.

CYTOMEGALIC INCLUSION DISEASE

This condition, caused by cytomegalovirus (CMV), is the most common of the congenital infections. The incidence ranges from 10 to 20 per thousand live births. Although CMV is transmitted from one person to another only through intimate contact, when one individual in a household has the disease, almost everyone there will become infected. One-half the women of early childbearing age show no immunity to the disease; by the end of the third decade of life, however, almost everyone has been infected. Fortunately, while there are probably many fetuses exposed to CMV in the uterus, few have obvious damage from the infection. The greatest risk to a fetus occurs with the first infection ￬f the mother. It appears that although women can be infected with CMV in successive pregnancies, the risk to the fetus is low.

While pregnant mothers with CMV usually show no symptoms, the disease may result in an intrauterine death or premature birth. Infants with general signs of congenital infection—low birth weight, jaundice, rash (petechiae), anemia, a large liver and spleen, and encephalitis—are checked for cytomegalic inclusion disease by isolation of cytomegalovirus and by blood tests. Congenital malformations include cerebral calcifications, small head (microcephaly), and small eyes. Ninety percent of newborns with CMV infection are asymptomatic at birth. Of these, some will later show signs of congenital infection, such as disease of the retina, deafness, and developmental delay.

Although antiviral drugs are being investigated, there is as yet no specific treatment for cytomegalic inclusion disease. Because CMV may be shed in body secretions and urine for several years after birth, individuals who have intimate contact with these infants should take proper precautions. Good handwashing after contact significantly lowers the risk of acquiring the infection. Pregnant women, however, should (if possible) avoid contact with these infants altogether.

HERPES

Herpes simplex is a virus which can produce devastating disease in the newborn. In the adult, the type I virus has typically been associated with the mouth, type II with the genital area. Both types, however, can be found in either location. At times, genital lesions in the mother are visible and may produce pain or other symptoms. At other times, the mother is without symptoms and the condition can be detected only through a culture of the virus. Herpes infection in the newborn is, properly speaking, neonatal rather than congenital; that is, although it is possible for it to be transmitted through the placenta, it is most often acquired during passage of the infant through the birth canal when the mother has active herpes in the genital region. While genital herpes tends to exist in the latent form, it may reactivate periodically. It is at these times that the fetus is susceptible during the birth process.

The incidence of neonatal herpes infection ranges from .03 to 0.3 per thousand live births. It is anticipated when the baby has been exposed to active lesions during a vaginal delivery, and it is diagnosed in the infant by isolation of the virus and other laboratory tests. Typically, the newborn does not show signs of infection until five to nine days after birth. There are two types of neonatal herpes infection: **(1)** a mild disease of the skin and the mucous membranes of the mouth and eye and **(2)** a severe, generalized form which involves all organs of the body, including the brain. Many infants with the latter will die. Survivors may suffer severe aftereffects, such as microcephaly, disease of the retina, intracranial calcificatins, seizures, and developmental delay. Infants with neonatal herpes may therefore have significant central nervous system damage requiring intensive educational and therapeutic services.

Herpes infection is now being treated in the newborn period with antiviral drugs. While these appear to effectively reduce the number of deaths from the disease, severe brain damage often occurs, even with treatment. The real answer is prevention. Because herpes simplex is becoming an increasingly common venereal disease, it is important that active herpetic lesions of the genital region be identified during pregnancy. If active lesions are present at the time of delivery, a cesarean section is recommended prior to or shortly after the bag of water ruptures. Presumably, infection can be prevented by delivering the fetus before it passes through the birth canal and comes into contact with the infective herpetic lesions.

Occasionally, surviving infants may have a periodic herpes skin rash. Pregnant women and other high-risk individuals should avoid contact with these infants when lesions are active. When the lesions are crusted over or absent, the child is not likely to be infectious. Intermittent services may be rendered at these times or even during periods of active lesions—provided gloves and good hand-washing techniques are used.

Cystic Fibrosis

David P. Schor, M.D.

DESCRIPTION

Cystic fibrosis (CF) is a common and generally fatal disorder of childhood characterized by the production of abnormal mucus, progressive lung damage, and impaired absorption of fat and protein. Individuals with CF become less able to exercise and have frequent respiratory symptoms, such as coughing and wheezing. They often require hospitalization and treatment with various medications and therapies aimed at reducing the ill effects of the disease and lengthening the life span.

CAUSE

CF is transmitted by autosomal recessive inheritance; that is, both parents must be carriers. Together they have—with each pregnancy—a 25 percent chance of producing a child with this condition.

INCIDENCE

Among Caucasian children, cystic fibrosis is the most common of the inherited chronic diseases, affecting one in every two thousand births. It is much less common among other racial groups.

DETECTION

Signs of cystic fibrosis include chronic lung disease, increased salt concentration in the sweat, and decreased release of certain digestive enzymes by the pancreas. Certain abnormalities revealed on X-rays or during a physical examination may also indicate the presence of CF; for example, about 10 to 15 percent of children with CF have intestinal blockage at birth. It is usually possible to detect the condition in asymptomatic individuals through a properly performed "sweat test." Very young infants may not produce the volume of sweat necessary for this procedure, however, and it is sometimes necessary to repeat the test as the infant grows older.

Carriers manifest no symptoms and cannot be detected reliably by available tests.

COURSE

CF may manifest itself in different ways at different ages. There may be intestinal blockage at birth, failure to grow (without any other symptoms), or respiratory problems, which eventually become the predominant symptoms. Chronic cough, wheezing, and recurring pneumonias begin weeks to years after birth and progress to blockage of air flow to parts of the lungs. The resultant reduction in oxygen to the body puts the heart under increasing strain. Prolonged and repeated lung infections, which are common despite intensive use of antibiotics, inhibit oxygen delivery even further. There is risk of lung collapse and massive bleeding into the lungs. The average life expectancy for individuals with CF is currently around 20 years. Death is usually a result of pulmonary complications.

Children with CF often fail to grow properly. Most require enzyme supplements to help them digest proteins and fats. On rare occasions, they may develop diabetes, liver disease (cirrhosis), or a sudden expulsion of part of the bowel beyond the anus (rectal prolapse).

ACCOMPANYING HEALTH PROBLEMS

For persons with cystic fibrosis, the lung symptoms are the most disabling, the heart symptoms the least reversible, and the digestive tract abnormalities the easiest to treat. Intensive treatment of undernutrition—giving substantial nutrients intravenously for several weeks, for example—may significantly improve growth and well-being for a period of several months.

MEDICAL MANAGEMENT

Individuals with cystic fibrosis generally receive chest physical therapy in order to loosen secretions that block lung airways; they also take vitamin supplements, enzymes (to assist in proper digestion), and antibiotics (to treat infections). Specific mineral supplements may also become necessary as the condition progresses.

IMPLICATIONS FOR EDUCATION

Cystic fibrosis is an incurable disease that produces increasing disability with time. The rate of this progression varies significantly with different individuals. For example, symptoms may be minimal in one five-year-old with CF and severe in another.

While exercise intolerance and heightened susceptibility to infection may occur in preschoolers, these are not common. Also less likely with this age group is the need for medications or physical therapy away from home.

Children with CF are susceptible to catastrophic medical problems, such as bleeding into the lungs (pulmonary hemorrhage). Most, however, have a gradual rather than sudden decline in health. Clinic visits and hospitalizations become more frequent with time; and as the disease worsens and death approaches, the family and child are likely to be under significant emotional stress.

SEE ALSO

Failure to Thrive, Genetics, and *Growth and Nutrition*

Defects in Brain Development

James A. Blackman, M.D.

Although alterations in brain development can result from a variety of genetic and metabolic diseases, this discussion will cover only major structural defects that can occur during embryonic and fetal life. Such congenital malformations of the nervous system comprise a spectrum of disorders ranging from anencephaly, a lethal condition, to microscopic alterations in brain structure, which are generally compatible with life but may cause anything from mild learning disorders to severe mental retardation.

ANENCEPHALY

Evident at birth, anencephaly is characterized by the absence of the cerebral hemispheres and the overlying bones of the skull. Infants with this condition are usually either stillborn or they live only a few days.

HYDRANENCEPHALY

With hydranencephaly, the cerebral hemispheres are absent, and the space is filled with fluid. At birth the infant may look normal; however, if a light is held next to the head in a dark room, much of the fluid-filled skull will illuminate. The brain stem, responsible for the basic processes of life (such as breathing), is well formed and operational. Without higher cortical functioning, however, there can be no voluntary motor or intellectual development. Also, seizures may occur. These infants often die before reaching one year of age, though a few survive beyond that time in a very primitive state of functioning.

HOLOPROSENCEPHALY

Among the numerous defects that may occur during the process of differentiation and growth of the cerebral hemispheres is holoprosencephaly. Children with this condition have a single cerebral sphere instead of the usual paired structures. As a result, they have severe motor and mental defects and rarely survive past infancy. Some children with holoprosencephaly have been found to have chromosomal abnormalities.

AGENESIS OF THE CORPUS CALLOSUM

Normally, the two cerebral hemispheres are connected by a midline fiber tract called the *corpus callosum*. The child in whom this structure fails to form may have difficulty transferring information from one cerebral hemisphere to the other. This may become more problematic with age, as it becomes necessary to process information requiring input from both hemispheres. In some individuals, agenesis of the corpus callosum is associated with other severe central nervous system malformations which may cause seizures, developmental delay, and hydrocephalus. This disorder is typically diagnosed using computerized axial tomography (CAT).

PORENCEPHALIC CYST

A cyst-like expansion of the lateral ventricle, a fluid-filled space in the brain, can result from a defect in the development of the cerebral mantle (cortex) or from local damage to the brain during fetal life or early infancy. Depending on the size and location of the cyst, a child may have motor, sensory, or visual defects. If the cyst is in one hemisphere only, these problems are evident on the opposite side of the body. For instance, a child with a left porencephalic cyst might have muscular stiffness (spastic hemiplegia) on his right side.

ENCEPHALOCELE

A malformation which occurs very early in the development of the nervous system is encephalocele, a condition similar to myelomeningocele in that there is a defect in the skull through which the brain, brain covering (meninges), or both extend. This defect is usually at the back of the head but may occur in other parts of the skull as well. Unlike other defects in brain development, encephalocele can usually be repaired surgically— unless there are other major malformations.

Encephalocele may be accompanied by hydrocephalus, which necessitates a shunt. If only the meninges protrude through the skull, there is a 60 percent chance the infant will have normal intelligence and motor function. If the brain is involved also, chances for normal intelligence drop to 10 percent.

MICROCEPHALY

Developmental abnormalities or destructive processes in the fetus or newborn may result in poor growth of the entire brain, a condition which is not treatable. A head circumference that is less than two standard deviations below the mean suggests abnormality; one that is three or more standard deviations below is a clear indication. Causes for microcephaly include recessive inheritance, chromosomal abnormalities, certain teratogens (e.g., radiation, alcohol), intrauterine infections (e.g., rubella), anoxia at birth, and severe malnutrition.

MEGALOCEPHALY

With this rare condition, there is excessive brain growth resulting in unusually rapid enlargement of the head. The growth is due to an increase in supportive tissues rather than an increase in the brain cells themselves. Megalocephaly must be differentiated from hydrocephalus and certain metabolic diseases which also cause excessive enlargement of the head. Severe mental deficiency is common.

SEE ALSO

Computerized Axial Tomography, Hydrocephalus, Myelomeningocele, Neuroanatomy, and *Teratogens*

Dental Disease

Arthur J. Nowak, D.M.D.

DESCRIPTION

Dental disease is an aggregate of conditions found in and around the mouth which may be due to heredity, congenital defects, infectious diseases, trauma, and neglect. The most frequently encountered dental diseases are cavities (caries), gum (periodontal) disease, and improper contact of upper and lower teeth and jaws (malocclusion). Also prevalent among children with developmental disabilities are enamel and dentin irregularities and fractured teeth.

CAUSE

The cause of dental disease varies with each condition. The two most prevalent conditions, cavities and gum disease, are brought about by the action of bacteria on carbohydrates and other substances. This metabolic activity produces acids and toxins in the plaque which, when allowed to remain in the mouth for a period of time, demineralize the enamel, producing cavities.

Similarly, toxins irritate the tissues around the teeth, causing inflammation and swelling of the gums (gingivitis). If allowed to continue, this disease progresses to the bone around the teeth (at which point it is referred to as periodontitis). Further loss of bone leads to loss of teeth.

Improper contact of the upper and lower teeth and jaws can result from (1) skeletal discrepancies between the upper and lower jaws, (2) discrepancy between tooth size and available space, (3) the loss of teeth due to cavities or gum disease, or (4) increased pressures on the teeth and jaws due to sucking habits or neuromuscular abnormalities.

Fractured teeth are usually caused by trauma, such as with falls or foreign objects striking the mouth. Occasionally, fractures result from pressure on teeth which have been previously weakened by cavities or enamel and dentin deficiencies.

INCIDENCE

The incidence of dental disease varies. It is uncommon to find a child who is totally free from one of the dental/oral conditions. With a few exceptions, cavities are no more prevalent among disabled than nondisabled children. They *are* more prevalent, however, in populations which are not exposed to fluorides. At least one-fourth of the two-year-olds and two-thirds of the three-year-olds in this group have some cavities. Children who have been on fluorides since birth, on the other hand, are commonly cavity-free.

Lengthy feedings also affect the incidence of cavities. Nursing caries—decay of the primary upper front teeth and first primary molars—are found in infants and very young children whose nursing sessions have been prolonged, especially those who have been put to sleep with a bottle.

The overall prevalence of gum disease is as high as 90 to 95 percent. (Fortunately, most of the gum disease found in children is of the mild variety caused by plaque and food debris from improper toothbrushing.) The prevalence among children with developmental disabilities is even higher, possibly a result of significantly poorer oral hygiene. Among children with Down syndrome, the prevalence of gum disease is very high and the incidence of cavities very low. There is, to date, no explanation for this finding.

Approximately 50 percent of the children who are on phenytoin (Dilantin) for treatment of convulsive disorders may develop gum overgrowth (gingival hyperplasia).

The prevalence of improper contact of upper and lower teeth in children with developmental disabilties is difficult to estimate. In normal populations, 30 percent of people have a receding lower jaw (Class II, or retrognathic, type of malocclusion); around 5 percent exhibit a protruding lower jaw (Class III, or prognathic, type). Studies have shown that as many as 90 percent of children with neuromuscular disorders have a malocclusion. Anterior open bites—when the top teeth overlap the bottom less than the normal 30 to 50 percent—are commonly found in children with developmental disabilities. This may be partially due to the higher incidence of tongue thrusting and mouth breathing or to weak oral-facial musculature.

DETECTION

Occasionally, an inquisitive parent may notice a mark or a defect in the mouth or on the teeth and bring it to the attention of a dentist. Generally, though, the child is first taken to the dentist because of pain or trauma, to fulfill a school entry requirement, or at the recommendation of a physician. Too frequently, by that time the child already has a dental problem.

It is now recommended that children with developmental disabilities, along with other high-risk children, be seen by a dentist within six months after the first tooth erupts. This way, in addition to examining the teeth and mouth, the dentist can initiate a comprehensive preventive dentistry program which should reduce or eliminate dental disease.

COURSE

Dental disease, especially cavities and gum infections, is progressive. Its effect on both the primary and permanent teeth can be devastating. If primary teeth are lost prematurely, the consequences can include decreased eating ability, interference with speech development, loss of space for the developing permanent teeth, and, possibly, temporomandibular joint disorders.

Cavities that progress to involve the pulp can lead to considerable pain as well as to infection that can rapidly involve many areas of the oral-facial complex. Gum disease does not advance as rapidly in children as it does in adults. Unfortunately, this fact has led to the erroneous notion that it affects only adults and is very unlikely in children.

Fractured teeth which are not properly treated can lead to pulp death (necrosis), with the possibility of infection and tooth loss. Teeth with enamel irregularities are not only aesthetically unpleasing, they are also more likely to fracture or develop cavities.

ACCOMPANYING HEALTH PROBLEMS

Clinical experience suggests that children with serious dental problems may have other health problems as well. Difficulty in chewing frequently leads to a compromised diet, one usually made up of high-calorie carbohydrates at the expense of fresh fruits and vegetables and protein-rich foods. Children with severe dental problems have a high incidence of ear, nose, and throat problems, which often disappear once the dental problems are resolved.

Some reports suggest that children with severe malocclusions may also exhibit temporomandibular joint dysfunction. Too, as mentioned earlier, there seems to be a high correlation of anterior open bite with mouth breathing and tongue thrusting.

DENTAL MANAGEMENT

Managing dental disease in children depends upon making parents aware of the importance of good dental care. Also essential are early examination and the initiation of a comprehensive preventive dentistry program. High-risk children should be seen initially by the dentist six months after the first tooth erupts. At this time, parents will be counseled regarding dental development, methods of cleaning the teeth and massaging the gums, modification of the diet, and optimal use of fluorides.

Cleaning the teeth

Teeth should be brushed as soon as they begin to erupt. A convenient method is to place the infant in a cradle developed by two adults sitting in a knee-to-knee position: one stabilizes and keeps the child involved while the other wields a small multitufted soft brush that effectively cleans the teeth and massages the gums. Toothpaste is not necessary for cleaning and may cause gagging. This cleaning should take place at least once a day, preferably before sleep. As the child grows and becomes more involved in the cleaning process, adults should continue to evaluate and reinforce his efforts.

Recommended Position for Cleaning Child's Teeth

Diet

Diet plays a major role in the origin and development of dental disease. A child's diet should be monitored, with restrictions placed on foods—including snacks—that are adhesive or slowly dissolving and on foods which have a high table sugar (sucrose) content.

Fluoridation

Fluoridating community water has brought a 48 to 70 percent reduction of cavities in children with lifelong exposure. In communities where water is not fluoridated, children should be given fluoride supplements. Professionally applied fluorides are also recommended either annually or semiannually, depending on the child's dental needs. (The suggested dosages may have to be adjusted for the child's disability, dietary habits, and disease patterns.)

SUPPLEMENTAL FLUORIDE DOSAGE SCHEDULE
(Adjusted allowance in mg. F/day)

Age in Years	Concentration of fluoride in water (ppm)		
	Less than 0.3	0.3 to 0.7	Greater than 0.7
Birth to 2	0.25	0	0
2 to 3	0.50	0.25	0
3 to 14	1.00	0.50	0

Approved by the Council on Dental Therapeutics of the American Dental Association and Committee on Nutrition of the American Academy of Pediatrics.

The use of pacifiers

Although thumb and finger sucking can have a profound effect on the growth and development of the teeth and jaws, it is common for infants and young children to require additional sucking. Whether a pacifier is less detrimental than finger and thumb sucking to growth and development is still being investigated. Some professionals feel that a pacifier is preferable, partly because it can be withdrawn at the appropriate age.

Even with the most comprehensive preventive dentistry program, dental disease may still occur. Generally, all of the restorative techniques that have been developed are available for use with all children. Unfortunately, children with developmental disabilities may be more difficult to manage in a dental setting. Some may be given general anesthesia, while others may need to be sedated with drugs or stabilized with restraints. Management problems make it even more important that these children visit the dentist frequently in order to intercept problems early and to avoid extensive and complex treatment.

IMPLICATIONS FOR EDUCATION

Children with dental disease may present many problems in the educational setting:

- Pain from the mouth may cause difficulty in properly chewing food. A compromised appetite may lead to either reduced food intake or a modified diet.
- Missing teeth, especially in the anterior segment, can interfere with the proper placement of the tongue and lips, possibly interfering with the speech mechanism.
- Decayed and missing teeth may interfere with social acceptance because of compromised aesthetics and smell.

- Untreated dental disease can lead to pain and discomfort. Children may not be able to cope with pain or understand its management; they may be hyperactive or have decreased attention spans.
- Dental disease may require considerable professional attention, taking time away from the classroom.

Additionally, educators must be careful that children with neuromuscular problems or with uncontrolled convulsive disorders are properly supervised to avoid trauma to the face, mouth, and teeth. During feeding, utensils must be carefully managed so that the child will not inadvertently bite down on them and damage teeth or soft tissues.

Every effort should be made to reduce the frequency of foods, including snacks, that are high in sucrose. These foods have a tendency to remain on the teeth, and the subsequent production of acids may cause cavities.

The classroom can be an excellent environment for teaching proper toothbrushing skills. The physical and/or occupational therapist can utilize the procedure as a means of developing a systematic approach to personal hygiene and task orientation.

Down Syndrome

James A. Blackman, M.D.

DESCRIPTION

Down syndrome, sometimes called trisomy 21 or, less acceptably, mongolism, results from one of the most common chromosomal abnormalities in humans—the presence of an extra chromosome, or extra part of a chromosome, in each cell of the body. This anomaly causes the physical and developmental features of Down syndrome:

- Congenital heart disease
- Mental retardation
- Small stature
- Decreased muscle tone (hypotonia)
- Hyperflexibility of joints
- Speckling of iris (Brushfield spots)
- Upward slant to eyes
- Extra fold at inner corner of eyes (epicanthal folds)
- Small oral cavity, resulting in protruding tongue
- Short, broad hands with single palmar crease (simian crease)
- Wide gap between first and second toes

The presence and degree of the above characteristics vary with each child. Many other features are associated with Down syndrome, and some of those listed above may be found in children without this condition.

CAUSE

The various physical and mental abnormalities associated with Down syndrome are caused by a genetic imbalance: there is an extra chromosome in all or most cells of the child's body. Normally, every cell of the human body except for the gametes (sperm or ova) contains 46 chromosomes, which are arranged in pairs. With Down syndrome there is one extra, or 47 chromosomes. There are three processes by which this anomaly can occur:

Nondisjunction

Chromosomal pairs are numbered according to size (numbers 1 to 22, plus two sex chromosomes). Failure of the #21 pair to separate accounts for 95 percent of the cases of Down syndrome. This nondisjunction of the #21 pair takes place prior to conception—during the formation of the sperm or ovum in the parent. The abnormal gamete then joins with a normal gamete at conception to form a fertilized egg with three (a *trisomy* of) #21 chromosomes. (This may also occur during the first cell division after conception.) This type of Down syndrome is usually sporadic and has a recurrence rate of 1/2 to 1 percent.

Chromosome Pattern (Karyotype) of a Body (Somatic) Cell in a Male with Down Syndrome. *Notice the extra #21 chromosome.*

Translocation

In 4 percent of the cases of Down syndrome, the extra #21 chromosome is attached (translocated) to another chromosome (usually #14, 15, or 22). About half the time, this type of Down syndrome is inherited from a parent who is a "carrier." The risk of recurrence is therefore much higher than with nondisjunction.

Mosaicism

In another 1 to 2 percent of cases, the abnormal separation of #21 chromosomes occurs sometime after conception. All future divisions of the affected cell result in cells with an extra chromosome. Therefore, the child has some cells with the normal number of chromosomes and other cells with an extra chromosome. The extent to which the child has the features of Down syndrome depends on the percentage of body cells with the extra #21 chromosome. The recurrence risk for this type of Down syndrome is not significantly different from the risk in the general population.

No specific cause for these chromosomal abnormalities has been identified. However, the risk of having a child with Down syndrome increases with advancing maternal age. (Amniocentesis is commonly available for prenatal diagnosis.) In one-third of the cases, the extra chromosome comes from the father.

INCIDENCE

Down syndrome occurs in approximately 1 in 600 to 800 live births, a figure that does not take into account the large number of affected fetuses which are aborted spontaneously. All races are affected equally. Incidence increases with the age of the mother; one study estimates the rate for women of 40 years of age at 1 per 110 live births.

DETECTION

The physical characteristics of Down syndrome usually make it evident at birth. The diagnosis is confirmed by growing certain white blood cells in the laboratory and photographing them as they undergo cell division. This chromosomal analysis, called a karyotype, can also be done on fetal cells obtained by amniocentesis, making prenatal diagnosis possible. If the karyotype of an individual with Down syndrome reveals the translocation type, it is important to examine the karyotype of the parents to determine whether they are carriers.

COURSE

With medical and surgical intervention—the correction of heart defects, for instance—and with improved educational opportunities, the prognosis for children with Down syndrome has improved dramatically. Many survive beyond the ages of 50 or 60. The most significant improvements in their physical and mental development have resulted from deinstitutionalization and from training in self-help and work skills.

Children with Down syndrome tend to be hypotonic, that is, to have low muscle tone at birth, making them floppy and poorly coordinated; this improves with age, however. Overall growth is relatively slow, and final height is reached at around 16. Girls may menstruate and be fertile, but males are usually infertile.

Mental retardation, which is invariably associated with this syndrome, becomes more evident as the child grows older and IQ and social maturity tests include more items calling for abstract reasoning. Performance on adaptive behavior tests, on the other hand, usually improves. (This is true of mentally retarded children in general.)

ACCOMPANYING HEALTH PROBLEMS

Serious health problems which may accompany Down syndrome are congenital heart disease and blockage in the small intestine (duodenal atresia). Because these children have a lowered resistance to infection, they frequently have respiratory infections, runny nose (chronic rhinitis), and conjunctivitis. Also common are eye problems, such as crossing (strabismus) or refractive errors (e.g., farsightedness and nearsightedness), and mild-to-moderate hearing loss.

MEDICAL MANAGEMENT

To assure survival, major medical problems, such as congenital heart disease and duodenal atresia, require specialized medical and surgical treatment in infancy. After this, health problems associated with Down syndrome are relatively minor and are treated the same as they are with all children.

IMPLICATIONS FOR EDUCATION

While the degree of mental retardation accompanying Down syndrome varies from mild to severe, most affected children are in the moderate range. The retardation, coupled with low muscle tone, leads to delays in development which affect educational performance.

Infants with Down syndrome may seem passive and content to lie quietly, but in order to develop fully they need to be handled, talked to, and played with. They also benefit from exposure to music, colors, textures, movement, and the like. Simple toys and simple tasks reduce frustration and are therefore more conducive to growth. Self-help skills are harder for these children to learn and require constant practice to maintain.

Like all children, children with Down syndrome need discipline. Correction procedures are most effective when used to augment imitation and positive reinforcement.

As infants, these children eat slowly and tend to spit up a mouthful or two after feedings. This may cause them not to grow well when they are young. As they get older, however, many are prone to obesity; therefore, high-caloric snacks should be avoided, and regular exercise should be encouraged. Constipation, too, is common and may be handled with increased amounts of water, fruits, and roughage.

Respiratory infections are frequent, particularly in the very young, and may interrupt the educational process. Adequate humidity in the classroom may help alleviate stuffy noses and upper respiratory problems.

SEE ALSO

Approach to Syndromes, Congenital Heart Disease, Genetics, and *Mental Retardation*

Electroencephalo-graphy

David P. Schor, M.D.

The electroencephalogram (EEG) is a recording of the electrical signals produced by the brain. Electrodes placed on the scalp surface pick up electrical impulses of millions of nearby nerve cells and carry them to the EEG machine, where they are amplified and combined with signals from other areas of the brain surface. (Signals from deep within the brain are usually too weak to be recorded.)

Sites of Electrode Placement

The test causes no pain, though it may frighten the child, making sedation necessary. The normal EEG pattern for adults is not developed until late childhood, and correctly interpreting the EEGs of children—particularly those of newborns—requires specialized knowledge and experience.

The following readouts for a normal child of one month, one year, and four years illustrate how much EEG patterns change as the brain develops:

ONE MONTH

ONE YEAR

FOUR YEARS

Normal EEG Patterns at Different Ages

The EEG is the most useful laboratory test for children suspected of having seizure disorders. Various EEG patterns are associated with specific types of seizures. Some children who have seizure disorders, however, may have a normal EEG (although specialized techniques or placement of receiving electrodes sometimes reveals characteristic abnormalities in EEG patterns). Just as a seizure disorder may not be reflected in the EEG, an abnormal EEG does not necessarily mean there is a seizure disorder. About 15 percent of the population have EEG abnormalities which are not associated with clinically evident seizures.

NORMAL AT ONE YEAR

ABNORMAL AT ONE YEAR

Normal and Abnormal EEG Patterns

It is best to get an EEG just before and during sleep, the times when seizure patterns are likely to be most evident. For this reason, drugs are sometimes used to produce drowsiness.

Electroencephalograms are also useful in diagnosing brain malformations, tumors, abscesses, and pockets of blood—all of which alter the typical patterns. They are also useful in determining brain death by detecting the absence of electrical activity—a criterion used by some facilities to determine when to discontinue the use of life-support mechanisms.

Efforts have been made to derive additional information from EEG patterns using computers. For example, an individual's response to a repeated sound (auditory evoked response, or AER) can be assessed by sending certain EEG signals to a computer. This technique, which does not require cooperation by the child, may be useful in assessing hearing in children too young or too developmentally delayed to give reliable responses with other methods. A similar technique, which computes visually evoked responses (VERs), can be useful in assessing vision in very young or mentally retarded children. Another recently developed technique, called brain electrical activity mapping (BEAM), combines EEG data with a computer to produce a visual image of the brain's electrical activity.

SEE ALSO

Hearing Impairment, Seizure Disorders, and *Visual Impairment*

Encephalitis and Meningitis

Mark L. Wolraich, M.D.

Encephalitis and meningitis are infections which involve the central nervous system.

ENCEPHALITIS

DESCRIPTION

Encephalitis is an infection of the brain substance.

CAUSE

This condition is almost always caused by a virus, usually one that can cause infections of other tissues as well (e.g., mumps, influenza). For some unknown reason, in certain individuals the virus attacks the brain. Occasionally, there are epidemics of encephalitis caused by certain viruses, such as the eastern or western equine type. Mosquitoes carry these from birds and domestic and wild mammals to humans.

INCIDENCE

The incidence of encephalitis is hard to determine, since this condition is difficult to diagnose and therefore may go unreported. While any individual can be affected, this disease is more likely to occur in children. Some of the viruses cause encephalitic infections on a year-round basis; others, such as the mosquito-borne viruses, cause infections mainly during the summer months.

DETECTION

The different locations of the infection result in different symptoms. The initial symptoms of encephalitis include fever, vomiting, various alterations in brain function (confusion, dizziness, headache, drowsiness), and, if the disease is in its more advanced stages, seizures and coma.

Encephalitis is diagnosed primarily from the physical exam, though tests may be done to rule out other conditions.

COURSE

This condition is usually mild (except in the case of neonatal herpes simplex encephalitis). However, it may progress to coma and, in a very small percentage of children, death. Most children will recover without any aftereffects. A small percentage, however, may incur brain damage, resulting in some degree of mental retardation or learning disability. A rare, slowly progressive form of encephalitis, called subacute sclerosing panencephalitis, causes gradual, ongoing brain damage and, ultimately, death.

ACCOMPANYING HEALTH PROBLEMS

The primary health problem which can occur with encephalitis is brain damage. This may result in mental retardation, learning disabilities, and/or a convulsive disorder. Brain damage can also lead to blindness, deafness, hydrocephalus, hyperactive behavior, or paralysis.

MEDICAL MANAGEMENT

Generally speaking, there are no medicines for treating viral infections (though a drug has been used with some success with herpes virus infections). Therefore, in the case of encephalitis, treatment consists of controlling the symptoms until the infection subsides on its own. Fortunately, most viral infections are eventually cleared by the body's own defense mechanisms without any lasting effects.

IMPLICATIONS FOR EDUCATION

Most children who have had encephalitis have no long-lasting effects. Only those children who have incurred brain damage and resultant problems will require special instructional techniques.

MENINGITIS

DESCRIPTION
Meningitis is an infection of the covering (meninges) surrounding the brain and spinal cord.

CAUSE
Meningitis, like encephalitis, can be caused by a virus. More commonly, though, it is caused by bacteria. In the newborn period, when the mortality rate for this condition is highest, meningitis is usually due to organisms normally found in the intestinal tract and vagina of the mother and is acquired by the infant during passage through the birth canal. In children aged two months to three years, the cause is usually one of three organisms: *Hemophilus influenzae,* meningococcus, or pneumococcus.

INCIDENCE
The incidence of neonatal meningitis in full-term infants is 0.13 per thousand births. In preterm babies this figure increases 2.24 per thousand. Forty in every ten thousand children aged one month to three years are affected by *Hemophilus influenzae,* the leading cause of bacterial meningitis in this age group.

DETECTION
The signs and symptoms of bacterial meningitis vary with the age and development of the child. Signs and symptoms are likely to include a bulging soft spot (in the infant), fever, stiff neck, irritability, poor feeding, vomiting, and even seizures. The older child may complain also of headache. Meningitis is diagnosed by performing tests on spinal fluid, which is obtained safely and easily by a spinal tap (lumbar puncture). These tests include a culture of the spinal fluid to determine whether the infection is caused by a virus or bacterium, and if the latter, which type. This culture also indicates whether the disease can be treated with antibiotics, and if so, which ones.

COURSE
The course meningitis follows depends on which organism causes it. If the disease is due to a virus, the progression is similar to that of encephalitis, and the majority of children will recover on their own without any aftereffects. If, on the other hand, the meningitis is caused by a bacterium, it can result in severe brain damage or even death. Fortunately, bacterial meningitis is generally treatable with antibiotics; and if these are

administered early enough, it can be cured with no long-term effects. The younger the child and the longer the infection goes untreated (or inadequately treated), the greater the likelihood of serious long-term effects.

ACCOMPANYING HEALTH PROBLEMS

The primary health problem which can occur with meningitis is brain damage. Neonatal meningitis, usually bacterial, is associated with permanent neurologic damage in 30 to 50 percent of its survivors. These problems include hydrocephalus, mental retardation, blindness, hearing loss, motor disability, and abnormal speech patterns. There may also be perceptual difficulties, learning disabilities, and behavioral problems.

MEDICAL MANAGEMENT

If the meningitis is caused by a virus, treatment consists of controlling the symptoms until the infection subsides on its own, usually without any lasting effects. Bacterial meningitis, on the other hand, requires treatment with antibiotics effective in killing the specific bacteria involved. In order to reach the central nervous system in adequate concentrations, most antibiotics must be administered intravenously, at least in the early stages, and the child must be hospitalized.

IMPLICATIONS FOR EDUCATION

Special instructional techniques are required only with those children who have incurred brain damage and resultant problems, including mental retardation, learning disabilities, hyperactivity, hydrocephalus, deafness, and blindness.

SEE ALSO

Convulsive Disorders, Hearing Impairment, Hydrocephalus, Mental Retardation, and *Visual Impairment*

Failure to
Thrive

David P. Schor, M.D.

DESCRIPTION

Children who weigh significantly less than their peers or who gain weight at a slower-than-normal rate during infancy or early childhood are said to "fail to thrive."

Some children are normal but small due to hereditary factors. With others, small size is a sign of underlying problems: the body, for various reasons, either does not receive or cannot properly utilize the nutrients required for proper growth and development. If this malnutrition is prolonged, weight, height, and eventually head size (brain growth) are affected.

CAUSE

The reasons for failure to thrive may be organic or nonorganic or both. Organic causes include numerous disorders, especially central nervous system, cardiovascular, and digestive tract problems. For example, with chronic heart failure, the body has higher-than-normal caloric requirements. With cystic fibrosis, the intestines do not adequately absorb fats and proteins, and the child may fail to thrive despite apparently adequate food intake.

More common is nonorganic failure to thrive. In many regions of the world this is due mainly to poverty, ignorance, or inappropriate dietary and feeding practices. In the U.S. this condition is more often associated with neglect, emotional disturbances, or ignorance on the part of parents who are often themselves victims of poor parenting and ongoing stresses. Difficulties in parent-child relationships may result in feeding problems: parents may become impatient with the feeding process; children may refuse to be fed or they may even resort to vomiting. Some cases of failure to thrive involve chronic parental depression or other emotional problems. In other situations there is deliberate neglect, sometimes with accompanying physical abuse.

Failure to thrive is more common among children with developmental disabilities than among nondisabled children. For some developmentally disabled children, growth potential is limited despite adequate feeding practices and food intake. Children with certain chromosomal abnormalities, for example, grow poorly even with greater-than-normal amounts of food. On the other hand, children whose poor growth is due to difficulties with the mechanics of chewing and swallowing may catch up with their peers if they are given adequate nutrients by other routes (a gastrostomy tube, for instance). Some children with disabilities are difficult to feed because of temperament or feeding-time behaviors, common in all children, that lead to stress or conflict. Parents or other caretakers need help in eliminating some of these negative behaviors. At times, hospitalization or assessment by a team of professionals (nutritionists, occupational therapists, psychologists) may be required to sort out the factors responsible for poor growth and to devise a plan for treatment.

SOME CAUSES OF FAILURE TO THRIVE

Organic causes

- Central nervous system abnormalities
- Structural or neuromotor abnormalities of the alimentary tract (e.g., cleft palate, cerebral palsy)
- Gastrointestinal diseases (malabsorption syndromes)
- Congenital heart disease
- Endocrine disorders (e.g., growth hormone deficiency)
- Chromosome defects
- Kidney disease
- Chronic infections
- Malignancies
- Fetal alcohol syndrome

Nonorganic causes

- Inadequate nutrient intake
- Environmental stress
- Emotional deprivation
- Abuse and neglect

INCIDENCE

Failure to thrive is diagnosed in about 1 percent of hospitalized children. In nonhospital medical settings this figure is much higher.

DETECTION

Charts giving normal ranges for weight, height, and head size are consulted to determine whether a child is small for age and sex. A series of measurements of more than two standard deviations below the mean over a period of months suggests a diagnosis of failure to thrive. Once the condition has been identified, a thorough medical history and physical examination are necessary to find the cause. At times, hospitalization for observation and testing may be required. If there is no organic cause and the child's growth improves with adequate nurturance, the failure to thrive is diagnosed as nonorganic.

COURSE

The course of failure to thrive depends on the timing, cause, and treatment of poor growth. Children with early (occurring in the first year) or prolonged failure to thrive have poorer growth than do children who are malnourished at a later age or for briefer periods.

Delays in gross motor, social, and expressive language skills may accompany failure to thrive. It is sometimes difficult to determine when delays in development are due to failure to thrive or vice versa. When adequate nutrition is restored, improvements in growth usually occur before improvements in developmental skills.

ACCOMPANYING HEALTH PROBLEMS

With organic failure to thrive, the signs and symptoms of the underlying disease tend to predominate. For example, while patients with cystic fibrosis may grow poorly because of impaired digestion of protein and fats, the poor growth is likely to be obscured by the more obvious symptoms of CF, such as coughing, wheezing, and frequent pneumonias.

Children with nonorganic failure to thrive often do not have regular checkups or adequate immunization. They are therefore more likely to have untreated medical problems, such as iron-deficiency anemia or impetigo.

IMPLICATIONS FOR EDUCATION

Undernourished children are at risk for learning problems, including mastery of gross motor skills—especially if the malnutrition is severe or prolonged or if it occurs within the first year of life. Children with significant organic failure to thrive during infancy may have reduced abilities in attention and memory. Children with nonorganic failure to thrive sometimes have difficulties with expressive language and social skills; they may have poor listening and attending skills as well.

A comprehensive interdisciplinary assessment of the child's strengths and weaknesses in cognition, academic tasks, language, social skills, and physical capacity, together with an understanding of the child's environment, helps enable teachers and families to design a program suitable for individual needs. Consultation may be necessary concerning specialized feeding techniques, behavior modification, or dietary manipulation.

SEE ALSO

Child Abuse and Neglect, Cystic Fibrosis, and *Growth and Nutrition*

Fetal Alcohol Syndrome

Frederick R. Schultz, M.D.

DESCRIPTION

Fetal alcohol syndrome (FAS) is a constellation of abnormalities directly related to alcohol ingestion during pregnancy. The major characteristics of FAS include both prenatal and postnatal growth deficiency, delay of gross and fine motor development (often associated with mental retardation), and congenital malformations, some of which result in a characteristic facial appearance.

CAUSE

FAS results from direct exposure of the fetus to the teratogenic effects of alcohol during pregnancy. The exact mechanism by which alcohol damages the developing body tissues is not understood. (Genetic predisposition or poor nutrition—both of which often accompany alcoholism—may be important contributing factors as well.) Since such organs as the brain and the heart are formed during the first trimester, it is clear that the consumption of alcohol during early pregnancy is cause for major concern. Alcohol can injure the fetus throughout the entire pregnancy, however.

There is at present no established amount of alcohol which a pregnant woman can consume without risk to her unborn baby.

INCIDENCE

Incidence rates for FAS vary, ranging from three to six cases per thousand live births. It has been estimated that between 50 and 75 percent of infants born to chronically alcoholic women may be affected with FAS.

DETECTION

Although some children with FAS can be diagnosed in the newborn period, affected children are often not identified until later in infancy or childhood. Presumably, many children with FAS are not identified at all.

ACCOMPANYING HEALTH PROBLEMS

Children with FAS are usually small at birth and continue to grow poorly. In addition, they often have delays in motor and mental development—FAS is one of the most common known causes of mental retardation—and they may exhibit behavior problems, such as hyperactivity. Physical abnormalities associated with this syndrome include small head, eyes, and mouth, as well as droopy eyelids, a wide space between the nose and upper lip, a thin upper lip, and occasional cleft palate and congenital heart disease.

COURSE

The physical, cognitive, and behavioral difficulties that the vast majority of these children have are often compounded by a poor home environment; the parents commonly have alcohol-related and other personal problems which prevent them from giving appropriate stimulation and nurturance. In many instances, the affected child is removed from the home environment. For some children, unfortunately, this means residing for short periods of time with several foster families rather than being raised in a single, long-term, stable setting.

IMPLICATIONS FOR EDUCATION

Many children with FAS have cognitive limitations and behavior problems which require appropriate adjustments in educational programming.

The ability of the natural parents to provide appropriate care may be limited. On the other hand, if the child is removed from parental custody, the possible lack of a stable, continuing, supportive home may contribute significantly to behavior problems.

SEE ALSO

Approach to Syndromes and *Mental Retardation*

The Floppy Infant

James A. Blackman, M.D.

DESCRIPTION

The floppy (hypotonic) infant, somewhat like a rag doll, assumes atypical postures, has excessive range of motion of the joints, and offers little resistance to passive movement. With young infants, the prominent feature of floppiness may be less than the usual amount of movement; with older infants, it may be delayed onset of motor milestones.

CAUSE

Generalized floppiness is symptomatic of a number of abnormal conditions in various parts of the neuromuscular system—the brain, spinal cord, peripheral nerve, and muscle:

Location	Example conditions
Brain	Hypotonic cerebral palsy, trauma, malformations, metabolic diseases (e.g., Tay-Sachs disease), Down syndrome
Spinal cord	Spinal muscular atrophy (Werdnig-Hoffmann disease), poliomyelitis, spinal cord trauma
Peripheral nerve	Neuropathies, myasthenia gravis, botulism
Muscle	Muscular dystrophies, metabolic disorders, connective tissue disorders, glycogen storage diseases

DETECTION

Floppiness is usually detected in the following manner (assuming the child is relaxed):

- When the child is held with one hand supporting the abdomen, the head and legs droop.
- When pulled by the hands to a sitting position, the child exhibits poor grasp, little tension of the arm muscles, and significant head lag.
- The child offers little resistance when body parts are moved by the examiner. For instance, an arm that is moved may remain in the new position.
- There may be passive movement beyond the expected range for the child's age. It is sometimes possible, for example, to extend the knees beyond the neutral (straight) position. It may also be possible, when the child lies faceup on a table with the hip and knee joints flexed, to spread the legs to touch the knees to the table.

A Floppy Infant

Once floppiness has been noted and demonstrated, it is important to determine the underlying cause. This means looking at the child's history as well as performing a physical examination and other assessments.

History

To explore the possibility of an inherited disease, the parents are asked whether other members of the family have been similarly affected. Details about the pregnancy and birth are sought as well, since they may point to perinatal brain injury. Another important step in tracking down the cause of floppiness is determining whether or not it was present at birth and if it has diminished or increased with time.

Physical examination

Growth parameters, including head circumference, are assessed. A small head (microcephaly) is an important clue to diagnosis. Particular attention is paid to the neuromotor part of the physical examination, which includes a precise evaluation of muscle function, reflexes, movement, body structure, and gross motor level. Findings in other areas—the skin or bones, for example—may suggest syndromes or diseases of which floppiness is a component.

Other assessments

The physical examination may point to the need for further laboratory tests (e.g., measuring muscle enzymes), specialized X-ray techniques (e.g., computerized axial tomography), an electromyogram (EMG), or even a muscle biopsy.

Input from other professionals is helpful in determining whether the floppiness is an isolated problem or whether the child is delayed in all areas of development.

The following are two examples of how this approach may be used to confirm a particular diagnosis:

CASE #1

History	Physical exam	Test	Diagnosis
Floppy since birth, mother's age at time of birth: 42	Upslanted eyes, flattened back of head, simian creases, wide-space between first and second toes	Chromosome analysis	Trisomy 21 (Down syndrome)

CASE #2

History	Physical exam	Test	Diagnosis
Full-term baby, progressively floppy during early months of life	Muscle weakness, absent deep tendon reflexes, twitching of the tongue	Electromography (EMG), nerve conduction velocities (NCV)	Werdnig-Hoffman disease

COURSE

In cases of benign congenital hypotonia—that is, where the floppiness is an isolated problem without other evidence of neurological abnormalities—the child may eventually become completely normal. In most instances of floppiness, however, the course is dependent upon the underlying condition, which may stabilize and remain unchanged or become progressively worse, resulting in death.

IMPLICATIONS FOR EDUCATION

It is important that the "floppy" infant undergo a thorough medical investigation and that early intervention professionals are informed of the diagnosis, prognosis, and accompanying health problems.

Since the hypotonic child will have difficulty moving, the early stages of development which are dependent upon physical interaction with the environment may be impeded. It is therefore necessary to "bring the environment to the child." This may be done by periodically moving the child to different areas of the room, by putting the child in a semi-upright supported position for ease of visual contact, by making certain that toys are within reach, and by making special attempts at interaction. ("Floppy" babies are sometimes left on their own and therefore do not receive appropriate stimulation.)

The amount of physical activity which should be encouraged depends on the diagnosis. The health and educational team need to work together to devise an individualized plan of developmental intervention for the child. Updated information regarding the child's medical condition should be requested frequently and adjustments in this plan made accordingly.

SEE ALSO

The Neurological Examination

Genetics

James A. Blackman, M.D.
Elizabeth Thomson, R.N., B.S.N.

PRINCIPLES OF INHERITANCE

Many developmental disabilities—physical, mental, or biochemical—are inherited. The basic unit of inheritance—whether the trait is hair color, height, blood type, or a particular genetic disease—is the gene. There are thousands of genes, which come in packages called chromosomes. In the cells of man there are normally 46 chromosomes, arranged in pairs (22 pairs called autosomes and one pair called sex chromosomes). Egg and sperm cells (gametes) include half the genetic material, or twenty-three single chromosomes, of the parent, so that at conception the fertilized egg (zygote) contains twenty-three *pairs* of chromosomes.

Chromosome abnormalities are detected by arranging and examining the chromosomes of a single cell that is typical of the individual, such as a white blood cell. This procedure is called karyotyping.

The Chromosomes as They Appear During Metaphase—A Stage in the Cycle of Cell Division

The Individual Chromosomes after Being Cut out and Arranged Sequentially in Pairs by Size, Shape, and Banding Pattern. *This karyotype of a normal female has 22 pairs of autosomes and one pair of sex chromosomes.*

GENETIC CAUSES OF BIRTH DEFECTS AND MENTAL RETARDATION

Multifactorial disorders

By far the greatest number of birth defects are caused by an interplay of genetic and environmental factors. Some examples are cardiac malformation, cleft of the lip and palate, and myelomeningocele.

Chromosome abnormalities

With this type of inheritance, there is either too much or too little genetic information present. There may be either too few or too many chromosomes, or there may be chromosomes with a piece missing or an extra piece attached.

SOME CHROMOSOME ABNORMALITIES

Abnormality	Disorder
• Extra #21 chromosome	• Down syndrome (Trisomy 21)
• Extra #18 chromosome	• Trisomy 18
• Extra #13 chromosome	• Trisomy 13
• Girl with only one X chromosome	• Turner syndrome (45, XO)
• Boy with an extra X chromosome	• Klinefelter syndrome (47, XXY)
• Structural abnormality of the X chromosome	• Fragile-X syndrome
• Deletion of the short arm of one #5 chromosome	• *Cri du chat* syndrome

Single gene disorders

With this type of genetic disorder, the amount of genetic material present is adequate. However, within the chromosomes there is an alteration in the genetic material of either a single gene or a pair of genes.

TYPES OF SINGLE GENE DISORDERS

Inheritance Pattern	Characteristics	Examples
Autosomal dominant parents: A a (affected) — a a (normal) gametes: A a — a a children: A a A a a a a a affected 50% normal 50%	Disorders are caused by a single altered gene on one of the autosomes. Either parent may have the gene, or the disorder may be due to a new gene alteration (mutation). If one parent is affected, there is a 50 percent risk of having an affected child (male or female) with each pregnancy.	Achondroplasia Huntington disease Tuberous sclerosis Neurofibromatosis Stickler syndrome Myotonic dystrophy
Autosomal recessive parents: A a (carrier) — A a (carrier) gametes: A a — A a children: AA A a a A a a normal 25% carrier 50% affected 25%	Disorders are caused by a pair of altered genes on the autosomes. Both parents are carriers of the altered gene (though they are clinically normal). When both parents are carriers, there is a 25 percent risk of having an affected child (male or female) with each pregnancy.	Cystic fibrosis Galactosemia Limb-girdle muscular dystrophy Maple syrup urine disease PKU Sickle cell anemia Tay-Sachs disease
X-linked recessive carrier mother parents: X X (carrier mother) — X Y (father) gametes: X X — X Y children: X X X Y X X X Y carrier daughter affected son normal daughter normal son	Either parent may have the gene present on the X-chromosome. Since females have two X-chromosomes, in order to be affected they must have a pair of altered genes. If a woman has an altered gene on only one X-chromosome, she is a carrier (usually not affected) and has a 25 percent risk of having an affected son.	Duchenne and Becker muscular dystrophies Hemophilia Hunter syndrome Color blindness Lesch-Nyhan syndrome

Inheritance Pattern	Characteristics	Examples
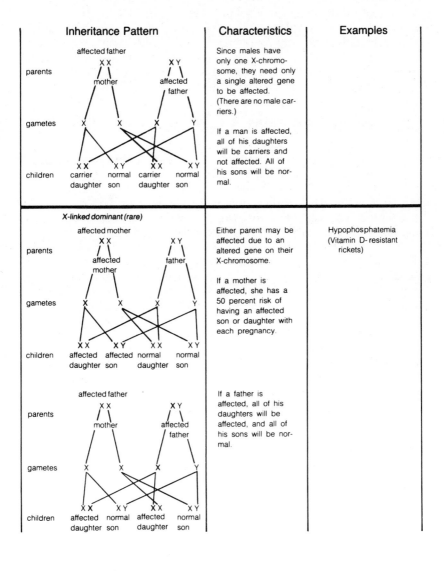	Since males have only one X-chromosome, they need only a single altered gene to be affected. (There are no male carriers.) If a man is affected, all of his daughters will be carriers and not affected. All of his sons will be normal.	
	Either parent may be affected due to an altered gene on their X-chromosome. If a mother is affected, she has a 50 percent risk of having an affected son or daughter with each pregnancy.	Hypophosphatemia (Vitamin D-resistant rickets)
	If a father is affected, all of his daughters will be affected, and all of his sons will be normal.	

DETECTION

There are three essential steps in evaluating a child who is suspected of having a genetic disorder: **(1)** outlining a detailed history of the health and development of individual family members; **(2)** examining the child thoroughly for signs and symptoms of specific genetic diseases; and **(3)** ordering specific laboratory tests, such as a chromosomal analysis (karyotype), X-rays, and biochemical studies of the blood and urine.

GENETIC COUNSELING

Families who are suspected of having a genetic disorder should be referred to a genetic counseling clinic. Genetic evaluation and counseling can sometimes aid in confirming or ruling out a specific diagnosis. Genetic counselors also help the family to comprehend the diagnosis, prognosis, and available medical management and to understand how the disorder is inherited, the risks of recurrence, and their reproductive options. In a genetic counseling clinic, families are encouraged to consider all available options and to choose what they feel is the appropriate course of action regarding the care of their child and further reproduction. Genetic counselors also try to help the family cope with the grief process and other problems that are inevitable when a child is diagnosed as having a birth defect or a genetic disorder. In addition, the counselors inform families about support groups, and, when appropriate, they make referrals to community agencies.

Families may have difficulty understanding all the information provided in a genetic counseling clinic, especially during a time of crisis. To make certain that the information is understood and that it is remembered, counselors see most families more than once. They also invite new questions as they arise and provide further counseling as other family members who may be at risk are identified.

SEE ALSO

Approach to Syndromes

Growth and Nutrition

James A. Blackman, M.D.

Infants and young children with developmental disabilities commonly do not grow as well as they should. Because proper nutrition is critical during early stages of growth—particularly growth of the brain—it must be monitored carefully in infancy and early childhood. Three physical measurements—weight, length, and head circumference—are plotted on standardized growth charts and used as gauges of nutritional adequacy. With each, the rate of growth is more important than the actual measurement at any given time.

WEIGHT

The average full-term newborn weighs approximately 3.4 kilograms (7.5 pounds). The average weight gain per day is 20 grams during the first five months and 15 grams per day throughout the remainder of the first year. Usually, an infant's weight doubles by five months and triples by one year.

The rate of growth slows during the second year, the average weight gain being about 2.5 kilograms (5 to 6 pounds). (This deceleration in rate of growth coincides with a corresponding decrease in appetite, which often worries parents.) In the next few years, annual weight gain is approximately 2.0 kilograms (4.5 pounds). By this time, children appear much leaner than they did as infants.

LENGTH

The average length at birth is 50 centimeters (20 inches). The infant grows around 25-30 centimeters (10 to 12 inches) during the first year, 12 centimeters (5 inches) during the second, and 6 to 8 centimeters (2.5 to 3 inches) each year thereafter.

HEAD CIRCUMFERENCE

Head circumference is one of the most important body measurements in that it provides an estimated rate of brain growth. A too rapid rate of increase in head circumference suggests hydrocephalus; a tapering off, potential problems with cognitive development. To find head circumference, a measuring tape is placed along the most prominent part of the back of the head and just above the eyebrows.

The average head circumference at birth is 34 to 35 centimeters. This increases rapidly (by approximately 12 centimeters) during infancy and then much more slowly (by 2 centimeters) during the second year. By the end of the first year the brain is approximately two-thirds of its adult size, and the number of its nerve cells is fixed. Further refinement continues, however, in the organization of brain function. Good nutrition, while not the only environmental factor affecting brain growth, is an essential prerequisite for optimal brain development.

WEIGHT

NATIONAL CENTER FOR HEALTH STATISTICS

Weight by age percentiles for girls aged birth-36 months.

GIRLS

WEIGHT

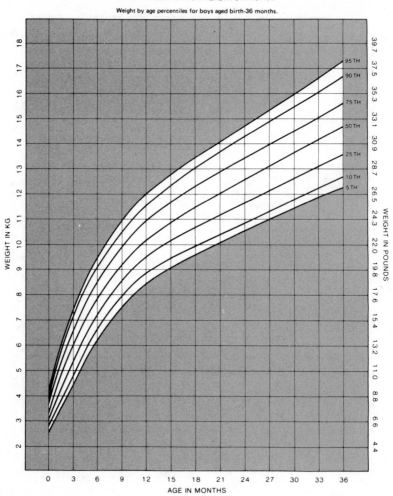

NATIONAL CENTER FOR HEALTH STATISTICS

Weight by age percentiles for boys aged birth-36 months.

BOYS

LENGTH

NATIONAL CENTER FOR HEALTH STATISTICS

Length by age percentiles for girls aged birth-36 months.

GIRLS

LENGTH

NATIONAL CENTER FOR HEALTH STATISTICS

Length by age percentiles for boys aged birth-36 months.

BOYS

HEAD CIRCUMFERENCE

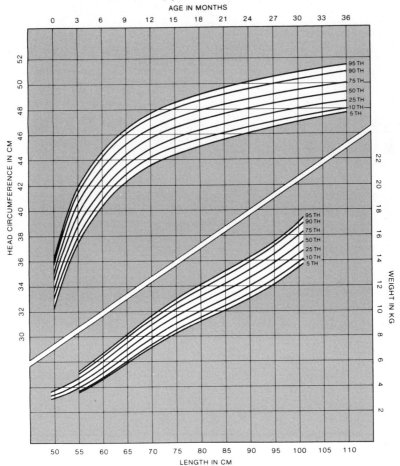

NATIONAL CENTER FOR HEALTH STATISTICS

Head circumference by age percentiles for girls aged birth-36 months.

Weight by length percentiles for girls aged birth-36 months.

GIRLS

HEAD CIRCUMFERENCE

NATIONAL CENTER FOR HEALTH STATISTICS

Head circumference by age percentiles for boys aged birth-36 months.

Weight by length percentiles for boys aged birth-36 months.

BOYS

PROBLEMS AFFECTING GROWTH

When a child is not growing at the expected rate, all growth parameters may be depressed, or there may be a discrepancy between the various parameters. Weight gain may be significantly below linear growth, for example. (Over 50 percent of children under three who were evaluated in a developmental clinic at The University of Iowa showed a weight gain which was low in comparison to their linear growth.)

In all cases of growth failure it is necessary to search for the causes. The following factors should be considered:

Nutrition

How much food is taken in by the child and how much is being retained? The child's usual food, fluid, and nutrient intake should be compared to the norms for children of the same length. Frequent variations in intake due to illness or other factors may account for poor growth. Also, certain dietary habits of parents (such as strict vegetarianism) may lead to the exclusion of important nutrients, as might the child's food preferences or problems with chewing or swallowing.

Parent-child interaction during feedings

Typical childhood behaviors such as food preferences, pickiness, and tantrums may interfere with or complicate intake. Oral-motor problems, too, often result in long and difficult feedings, causing stress for both parent and child. Growth may also be affected by how well the child indicates satiety and how well the caretaker responds.

Innate response characteristics of the child

Temperamental variations must be accounted for; some children are naturally placid in accepting food, others are resistant.

Physical growth expectations

It is true that some children have limited growth potential due to heredity or the nature of the disability. It is sometimes erroneously assumed, however, that because a child has a disabling condition (such as cerebral palsy) he cannot be expected to grow well. Such an assumption often masks the real and remediable problem underlying the poor growth: inadequate nutrition.

Structural, neuromotor, and sensory characteristics of the alimentary tract

In a large number of cases, intake of sufficient calories and other nutrients for proper growth and motor development is significantly impeded by neuromotor impairment. In other cases, poor growth is due to malabsorption and/or diarrhea.

Stamina

A problem which often goes unrecognized is that children may not eat well because of weakness. Among those whose food intake might be adversely affected by a lack of stamina are children with muscle diseases or congenital heart disease.

Failure to grow adequately may be the end result of any one or a combination of the above factors. Evaluation and treatment of poor growth requires input from a variety of professionals in medicine, psychology, nutrition, occupational therapy, and other disciplines. While some handicapped children's growth potential may be limited despite the best intervention, most can be helped to some degree.

SEE ALSO

Anemia and *Failure to Thrive*

Hearing Impairment

Gerri Kahn, Ph.D., CCC-A

DESCRIPTION

The normal ear responds to a wide range of sound intensities and frequencies. When hearing is impaired, this range of responsiveness to loudness and pitch is reduced.

Hearing impairment, which can range from mild to profound, is usually classified as one of two types: conductive or sensorineural. Conductive hearing loss occurs when there is a dysfunction in the outer or middle ear. Sensorineural hearing loss occurs when damage has been sustained by the inner ear or auditory nerve. If both a conductive and sensorineural hearing loss are present, the hearing loss is said to be mixed.

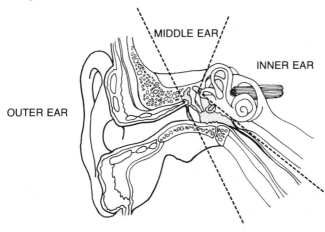

The Ear

With all types of hearing impairment, the perceived loudness of sounds is reduced (or even eliminated if the hearing loss is severe enough). Even sounds which are heard may not be heard clearly. With sensorineural and mixed hearing impairments, for example, speech sounds mushy or indistinct; one word may sound like another or like something that has no meaning whatsoever.

Hearing impairment may be unilateral (in one ear only) or bilateral (in both ears). Children with unilateral hearing impairment experience some difficulties, particularly in identifying the source of a sound (localization) and listening in a noisy environment. While they may have fewer problems than children with a bilateral hearing loss, it is important that they be identified, treated, if possible, and followed up.

CAUSE

By far the most common cause of conductive hearing impairment in children is middle ear disease (otitis media). Other causes include congenital malformations of the middle ear or a closing off of the ear canal by foreign bodies or wax (cerumen).

There are many causes for sensorineural hearing loss. Sensorineural impairment which is already present at birth may have been determined genetically, or it may be due to a maternal viral infection or a drug (particularly one ingested during the first trimester) which interferes with the normal development of the inner ear. Sensorineural impairment acquired during the birth process itself may be a result of lack of oxygen, head trauma, or other perinatal difficulties. That which is acquired months or years after birth may be caused by diseases (such as meningitis or mumps); it may also result from head trauma, exposure to certain drugs or extremely loud noises, or from a genetically determined condition that has its onset later in life.

INCIDENCE

It has been estimated that 25 to 65 percent of children under the age of two have had at least one ear infection, a condition which generally involves some conductive hearing loss.

Approximately three in every thousand children below the age of six have a greater-than-mild sensorineural hearing loss in both ears. If we include mild sensorineural loss, the incidence rate is increased 15 to 30 times.

DETECTION

Any child who fails to respond normally to sounds or who has delayed language or prelanguage behaviors should be evaluated for hearing impairment. Severe or profound hearing loss is easier to detect than mild or moderate hearing loss. With the former, the child rarely, if ever, responds to voices or environmental sounds. (It is, of course, crucial that all visual, tactile, and vibratory cues be eliminated when such judgments are made.) With mild or moderate hearing impairment, the child's responses to voices and environmental sounds are typically inconsistent, which often gives the erroneous impression that he hears when he wants to.

No child is too young for a formal hearing evaluation by an audiologist. While the techniques used and information derived may vary, some information about hearing can be obtained from a child of any age. The most common technique used with children under six months of age is observing their response—cessation of sucking, widening of the eyes, blinking, quieting, or turning of the head—to sounds of controlled intensities and frequencies.

From roughly six to twenty-four months, a visual reinforcer is often used. With this technique (visual reinforcement audiometry, or VRA), a flashing light or animated toy is used to reinforce a localization response (conditioned orientation reflex, or COR) to sounds of controlled intensities and frequencies.

Children around two to five years old are usually tested by a technique called conditioned play audiometry, whereby they engage in a play activity, such as putting a block in a box, each time a sound is heard.

The testing techniques used depend on developmental rather than chronological age. If the physical or mental condition of the child renders behavioral responses unobtainable or questionable, other techniques may be used to measure physiologic responses to auditory stimuli. It is necessary, however. to have behavioral-response corroboration of these results as soon as possible. One technique measures the acoustic reflex, that is, the contraction of muscles of the middle ear in response to intense sounds. If an exceedingly high intensity of sound is required for this contraction to occur, the child may have a severe or profound hearing loss. While researchers are currently attempting to be more precise at predicting degrees of hearing loss with this technique, it is still far from perfect. Another technique, called evoked response audiometry (ERA), monitors changes in brain waves when auditory stimuli are presented. Both muscle contractions and brain-wave responses, however, can be difficult to interpret in a child with neurological damage.

Once it has been established that the child has a hearing loss, the next step is determining the type (conductive, sensorineural, or mixed) and degree of hearing impairment. The hearing evaluation includes assessing middle ear air pressure and eardrum mobility with acoustic immittance measures (e.g., tympanometry). Abnormal results suggest a conductive component to the hearing impairment; normal results are typical of a pure sensorineural hearing loss.

There are two ways in which hearing sensitivity may be assessed; these can also help determine which type of impairment is present:

(1) Air-conduction testing—The child wears earphones from which sound is conducted down the ear canal, through the tympanic membrane and middle ear, and then to the inner ear. An impairment in any of these areas will cause a decrease in hearing sensitivity.

(2) Bone-conduction testing—The sound is conducted more directly to the inner ear by vibrating the skull, thereby measuring the sensitivity of the inner ear without the influence of the middle ear.

A comparison of hearing sensitivity as determined by air and bone conduction testing will reveal whether the hearing loss is conductive or sensorineural: If air and bone conduction tests show equally depressed sensitivity, the hearing loss is sensorineural. If sensitivity is depressed by air conduction but normal by bone conduction, the hearing loss is conductive. If sensitivity by bone conduction is depressed and sensitivity by air conduction is even more depressed, the hearing loss is mixed.

MANAGEMENT

All children with hearing impairment should have a medical evaluation (1) to look for signs of underlying diseases, some of which are treatable, and (2) to identify genetic factors for which counseling may be necessary.

In most cases of conductive hearing loss, successful medical or surgical intervention will return hearing to normal. A sensorineural hearing loss, on the other hand, is rarely medically or surgically treatable; it is almost always permanent. The primary management technique for sensorineural loss is amplification, usually with a hearing aid. With a mixed hearing loss, the conductive impairment is treatable while the sensorineural impairment is not.

Children of any age—even infants—can successfully use a hearing aid. It is basically a miniature, wearable public address system with a microphone to pick up the sound, an amplifier to make the sound louder, and a loudspeaker to deliver the amplified sound to the ear. There are several different styles of hearing aids. The two most commonly used with children are body-style hearing aids and behind-the-ear hearing aids.

CUSTOM-MADE
EARMOLD
(ACOUSTIC
COUPLER)

BODY-STYLE
HEARING AID

BEHIND-THE-EAR
HEARING AID

Two Styles of Hearing Aids

Unfortunately, a hearing aid cannot correct hearing in the same way that eyeglasses correct vision. While the hearing aid increases sound intensity, it does not completely clarify the sound perceived by the impaired inner ear. What's more, the hearing aid amplifies all sound, including undesirable noises. It is important, therefore, to have realistic expectations of amplification. While improvement is highly significant, hearing is still far from perfect.

IMPLICATIONS FOR EDUCATION

A conductive hearing loss can be treated medically to restore hearing. Until this happens, however, the child experiences significant hearing difficulty. Even though a conductive hearing loss is usually mild in degree, the problems it presents to a child during critical learning years can be severe. Several studies have shown—within the limitations of retrospective data—that older children with learning disabilities had a higher incidence of otitis media with probable conductive hearing loss during early childhood than did children with normal learning abilities. One reason may be the intermittent hearing loss which characterizes episodes of otitis media.

With a sensorineural hearing loss, even one that has been identified and amplified very early, the child has missed many early auditory experiences needed for prelanguage and language development; as a result there is at least some degree of language delay. In fact, because of the imperfections of amplification, learning in general can be a struggle. Usually, the more severe the hearing loss, the greater the difficulty. Most children with sensorineural hearing loss need the benefits of early intervention programs which are designed specifically for the hearing impaired. Special programming, or at least special supportive services, may be necessary throughout the school years.

An audiologist can offer valuable assistance, not only in evaluation, but also in developing appropriate communication techniques that will help maximize a child's learning. Common suggestions include: get the child's attention before speaking, face the child when speaking, speak naturally and do not overenunciate, and check the hearing aid several times daily to make sure it is turned on and that the batteries are working.

SEE ALSO
Middle Ear Disease

Hydrocephalus

Mark L. Wolraich, M.D.

DESCRIPTION

With hydrocephalus, there is an imbalance in the production and absorption of cerebrospinal fluid (CSF) in the body, resulting in an enlargement of the fluid-filled spaces in and around the brain. Left untreated, this condition can cause permanent brain damage.

CAUSE

Hydrocephalus is usually caused by blockage in the normal circulation of CSF.

(1) Cerebrospinal fluid is produced by blood vessels (choroid plexus) in the **VENTRICLES**.

(2) It flows through the **THIRD VENTRICLE,**

(3) then through the **AQUEDUCT OF SYLVIUS,**

(4) and into the **FOURTH VENTRICLE.**

(5) From the fourth ventricle, most of the cerebrospinal fluid flows into the **SUBARACHNOID SPACE** surrounding the brain, where it is reabsorbed into the bloodstream.

(6) The rest flows down the spinal cord and is reabsorbed there.

The Normal Flow of Cerebrospinal Fluid

Blockage of the normal flow of cerebrospinal fluid

If the normal flow is blocked, there is a backup of cerebrospinal fluid in the ventricles. The blood vessels go right on producing fluid, however, causing the ventricles to enlarge and put pressure on the brain. This buildup of cerebrospinal fluid causes the infant's head to grow large and the soft spots (fontanelles) to bulge. As the child grows older and the fontanelles close, the head will no longer expand. Untreated hydrocephalus can therefore result in brain damage.

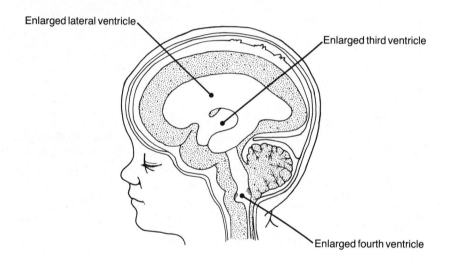

Enlarged lateral ventricle

Enlarged third ventricle

Enlarged fourth ventricle

Backup of CSF in the Ventricles

With a condition called noncommunicating hydrocephalus, the outflow of CSF from the ventricles is blocked. This sometimes occurs because the tube through which CSF normally passes from the third ventricle to the fourth is not properly formed (aqueductal stenosis). As a result, the fluid backs up in the lateral and third ventricles. Tumors and other congenital malformations, such as the Arnold-Chiari malformation (common among children with myelomeningocele) can also block the outflow of CSF from the ventricles.

With communicating hydrocephalus, CSF passes readily out of the ventricles but is blocked from being reabsorbed. This condition may result from meningitis, intraventricular hemorrhage in premature infants, or trauma.

Overproduction of cerebrospinal fluid

In rare cases of hydrocephalus, the channels for flow and absorption are open, but a tumor within the ventricular system produces more cerebrospinal fluid than can be reabsorbed; as a result, the head becomes enlarged.

INCIDENCE

The incidence of hydrocephalus in this country is approximately 0.8 to 1.6 cases per thousand children.

DETECTION

In children under one year of age, the first sign of hydrocephalus is usually a faster-than-normal increase in head size. As the condition progresses, the child's eyes may begin looking downward so that the white area above the pupil is prominent, a feature referred to as the setting-sun sign. The child may also become listless, irritable, and slow in developing. In older children, whose skulls can no longer expand, the symptoms are more acute; they include headache, vomiting, and coma.

Specialized X-rays called computerized axial tomography (CAT) scans can show the shape of the brain and dilated ventricles, thereby confirming the presence of hydrocephalus. In young children with open fontanelles, ultrasound can serve the same function.

COURSE

Left untreated, hydrocephalus produces further brain damage and may even be fatal. With proper medical and neurosurgical management, the majority of affected children will survive, though 60 percent will have significant intellectual and motor handicaps.

ACCOMPANYING HEALTH PROBLEMS

Some children with hydrocephalus also have seizure disorders. If hydrocephalus is accompanied by brain damage or brain malformation, mental retardation may be present as well.

MEDICAL MANAGEMENT

Hydrocephalus is usually treated with a ventriculo-peritoneal (VP) shunt, which helps lessen the pressure on the brain. A tube is inserted into the ventricles. This tube is connected to a one-way valve which lets the spinal fluid flow out of, but not back into, the brain. The valve is connected to another tube which is threaded just under the skin down into the cavity of the abdomen. The spinal fluid flows through the shunt and is reabsorbed by the blood vessels in the membranes surrounding the organs there. In rare instances, the tube in threaded into the heart rather than the abdomen; it is then called a ventriculo-atrial (VA) shunt.

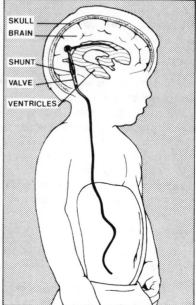

Ventriculo-Atrial (VA) Shunt   Ventriculo-Peritoneal (VP) Shunt

While this system usually works well, the insertion of the shunt may present some difficulties. First, the shunt hardware—a foreign object—provides a place for bacteria to multiply, sometimes resulting in infection. While this does not mean that special restrictions should be placed on the child, it does mean that a doctor should be consulted anytime the child is sick.

A second potential difficulty with a shunt is that, being mechanical, it is subject to clogging or other malfunctioning, which requires prompt attention. Irritability, vomiting, and fever are the most common signs of infection or shunt malfunction. Unfortunately, these are also the symptoms that children have with the usual childhood illnesses. This is why a physician's advice is always necessary.

Some children may outgrow the need for a shunt as circulation pathways expand, enabling them to maintain the delicate balance between the production and reabsorption of cerebrospinal fluid. This balance, however, may be upset by illness, making the shunt necessary to prevent recurrent hydrocephalus.

IMPLICATIONS FOR EDUCATION

While many children with hydrocephalus have no specific educational problems, others may have brain damage which results in motor, language, perceptual, or intellectual disabilities. The damage from the hydrocephalus is more likely to affect reasoning skills than rote memory. It is also likely to make these children hyperverbal. Extreme cases are characterized by the cocktail chatter syndrome—talking incessantly and with little meaning—or by echolalia—copying what other people say.

Children with hydrocephalus, like all children with disabilities, require a plan of individualized programming.

SEE ALSO

Computerized Axial Tomography and *Myelomeningocele*

Low Birth Weight

James A. Blackman, M.D.

A full-term baby usually weighs between 2,500 and 3,800 grams, or 5½ to 8½ pounds. A birth weight of less than 2,500 grams is considered low. A baby may have a low birth weight because of prematurity or intrauterine growth retardation or both. A premature (preterm) baby—one whose period of gestation was less than thirty-eight weeks—is small due to incomplete development. A baby who has suffered intrauterine growth retardation, on the other hand, may be small because of genetic makup or because of an unfavorable environment in the uterus. The causes, treatment, and outcome of these two conditions may be very different.

PREMATURITY

The usual gestational age—the length of time the fetus is carried in the uterus—ranges from 37 to 42 weeks. (Two techniques for determining gestational age are assessing the newborn's neuromuscular and physical characteristics and counting from the first day of the mother's last menstrual period.) Babies with a gestational age of less than 37 weeks are considered premature, or *preterm,* regardless of birth weight. While the exact cause of prematurity has not been determined, this condition has been associated with such varied factors as maternal trauma, teen pregnancies, poor prenatal care, and drug abuse.

A preterm baby may be physically normal—though immature—at birth, then develop serious problems during the postnatal period. These complications may, to varying degrees, damage the brain and other tissues, affecting future health and development:

Respiratory distress syndrome (RDS) (hyaline membrane disease)

Normally, the air sacs of the lungs are opened by the newborn's first breaths; they are kept open by a chemical coating called surfactant. If the premature infant does not produce enough surfactant, the lungs collapse after each breath. The result is too little oxygen in the blood and body tissues (hypoxemia) and a disruption of the acid-base balance (acidosis).

Infection

The child's immature defense mechanisms are sometimes unable to combat bacteria which are in the environment or which are introduced through intravenous lines, chest tubes for collapsed lungs, or other invasive equipment. This may result in an infection of the blood (sepsis) or an inflammation of the membranes surrounding the brain or spinal cord (meningitis).

Intracranial hemorrhage

There may be bleeding into the brain substance or, more commonly, around or into the fluid-filled chambers of the brain (peri- or intraventricular hemorrhage). This may result in the spastic type of cerebral palsy.

Malnutrition

Because many premature infants have difficulty tolerating oral feeding, they may suffer from temporary malnutrition. At times, these babies must receive their total caloric and fluid needs by intravenous feeding (hyperalimentation, total parenteral nutrition) or through a nasogastric tube.

Jaundice

Jaundice is a yellowish color of the skin and whites of the eyes caused by an accumulation of bilirubin in the body. Bilirubin, a product of the breakdown of red blood cells, is normally removed by the liver and excreted into the intestines. In preterm babies, the liver may not eliminate the bilirubin from the blood quickly enough. While moderate levels are usually inconsequential (except in sick or very premature babies), high levels may permanently damage the brain, particularly parts called the basal ganglia. Such damage, called kernicterus, may result in athetoid cerebral palsy.

Apnea

Apnea is a prolonged pause in respirations, often accompanied by a slowing of the heart rate (bradycardia) or a blue color to the skin (cyanosis). While this condition may occur in full-term infants, it is particularly common in those who are premature. Apnea must be distinguished from periodic breathing, typical in premature infants, in which a period of rapid breathing alternates with a short period (five seconds or so) of no breathing.

The sudden onset of apnea may indicate a serious illness, such as sepsis, meningitis, pneumonia, intracranial hemorrhage, or low blood sugar (hypoglycemia).

Physical stimulation is often adequate to reinitiate breathing. In the absence of serious illness, apnea is treated by environmental stimulation, such as a change in temperature or gentle rocking on a water bed. Medical therapy includes theophylline and caffeine; at times, cardiopulmonary resuscitation is necessary. Occasionally, babies are sent home from the hospital with apnea monitors, which sound an alarm when there is a prolonged period of no breathing.

Necrotizing enterocolitis (NEC)

Inflammation, and sometimes death, of intestinal wall tissue is a life-threatening complication, the exact cause of which is unknown (though it seems to be related to other problems which beset the preterm infant). In mild cases, conservative medical management is adequate; if a segment of the intestine dies, however, it must be removed surgically, and the shortened bowel may result in temporary—but prolonged—malabsorption of nutrients and diarrhea.

Patent ductus arteriosus

During intrauterine life, fetal circulation bypasses the lungs by means of a small blood vessel called the *ductus arteriosus*. This vessel normally closes at the time of birth. However, in some preterm infants or infants with heart defects, it may remain open, leading to enlargement of the heart and backup of blood in the lungs (congestive heart failure). In some cases, this vessel closes on its own or is closed by the administration of certain drugs; in other instances, it must be tied off surgically.

INTRAUTERINE GROWTH RETARDATION (IUGR)

For every gestational age there is a range of expected weights. An infant whose weight falls below the tenth percentile is considered small for gestational age (SGA). The SGA baby has usually suffered growth retardation in the uterus.

Although weight is used in defining intrauterine growth retardation, not all growth parameters are affected alike. Body weight is affected first, then body length, and lastly, brain size. For example, if the intrauterine insult occurs late in pregnancy, the infant's weight may be below the tenth percentile while its body length and head size are in the normal range. In contrast, if the cause for poor growth occurs during conception or early pregnancy, weight, length, and head size may all be affected equally.

Intrauterine growth retardation may be caused by genetic or inherited factors, or it may be due to an unfavorable environment in the uterus.

Genetic or inherited factors

Babies with congenital malformations or chromosomal abnormalities (e.g., trisomy-18 and Turner syndrome) are often small for gestational age. Too, certain families with no other developmental or growth difficulties have a tendency to produce small babies.

Unfavorable intrauterine environment

Extreme maternal malnutrition from deprivation or disease can affect the growth of the fetus. So can cytomegalovirus (CMV), rubella, and perhaps other infections as well. Intrauterine growth retardation is also associated with multiple births, cigarette smoking, high altitudes, drug addiction, alcohol abuse, toxemia, and hypertension.

Whereas the premature baby has had a favorable—though shortened—period of gestation, the baby who is small for gestational age has most likely had an unfavorable environment in the uterus. Depending on the nature, timing, and duration of the causal factor, organ systems may fail to develop normally in terms of size, structure, or function. For these reasons, the small-for-gestational-age baby often requires special care during the first few days of life. Insufficient oxygen in the blood at birth (neonatal asphyxia) tends to be more common and accentuated in these babies. The incidence of major congenital anomalies is also more common. SGA babies often have low blood sugar and may have too many red blood cells (polycythemia).

The baby who is small for gestational age may continue to grow poorly, not catching up as the preterm baby usually does. Whereas preterm babies often catch up during the second year of life, some SGA babies tend to remain smaller than average. In addition to poor growth, some studies have shown a higher than expected prevalence of developmental delay among SGA infants.

SEE ALSO

Congenital Infections and *Respiratory Distress Syndrome*

Mental Retardation

James A. Blackman, M.D.

DESCRIPTION

The American Association on Mental Deficiency defines mental retardation as "significant subaverage general intellectual functioning existing concurrently with deficits in adaptive behavior and manifested during the developmental period."

Despite the appropriate reluctance to apply the term *mental retardation* to children under three years old, it will be used in this chapter—keeping in mind that the various assessment techniques are limited in their ability to reveal this characteristic in the very young child.

CAUSE

When mental retardation is suspected, the child should have a thorough medical evaluation to try to determine the cause.

SOME CONDITIONS OR EVENTS ASSOCIATED WITH MENTAL RETARDATION

Period of development	Type of condition or event	Examples
Pre- and peri-conceptual	Metabolic disorders	Mucopolysaccharidoses Tay-Sachs disease
	Brain malformation	Encephalocele Hydranencephaly
	Neurocutaneous syndromes	Tuberous sclerosis Neurofibromatosis
	Chromosomal abnormalities	Down syndrome *Cri du chat* syndrome
Prenatal	Teratogens	Chemicals Radiation Alcohol
	Infection	Rubella Cytomegalovirus
	Fetal malnutrition	Mother with high blood pressure or kidney disease
Perinatal	Prematurity	Complications such as poor oxygenation of the brain and intracranial hemorrhage
	Metabolic abnor-malities	Asphyxia at birth Hypoglycemia
	Trauma	Misapplication of forceps
	Infection	Herpes simplex encephalitis
Postnatal	Infection	Meningitis
	Trauma	Automobile accident Child abuse
	Lack of oxygen	Near drowning Strangulation
	Severe nutritional deficiency	Kwashiorkor
	Environmental toxins	Lead
	Environmental and social problems	Psychosocial deprivation Parental psychiatric disorders

The physician considers systematically each of the above-mentioned causes for mental retardation. In the majority of cases—particularly when the retardation is in the mild-to-moderate range—the cause will not be identifiable. Even for most known causes there is no known treatment. And in the rare instance when the cause is both known and treatable, whatever brain damage has already occurred is irreversible. But despite these depressing odds, parents, educators, and anyone else who is concerned with the child's development and well-being are entitled to the assurance that no condition which might benefit from medical treatment has been overlooked. Also, since some causes may be genetic, proper identification may lead to counseling for parents and other family members regarding the risks of recurrence with future pregnancies.

In some cases, the diagnosis of conditions associated with mental retardation can be made either prenatally, through amniocentesis, or postnatally, through newborn screening programs intended to identify treatable metabolic diseases before permanent brain damage occurs.

The physician usually begins the evaluation with an investigation of the child's history. This includes details of the family tree and of the mother's pregnancy, labor, and delivery, along with information about the child's postnatal period and childhood illnesses or accidents.

A physical examination follows, with attention to signs which may suggest a specific diagnosis, such as peculiar facial features, skin pigment, or urine odor. By this time, many possible causes should be eliminated. Laboratory and radiologic procedures are then used either to narrow the possibilities or to pinpoint the diagnosis.

INCIDENCE

Because the label *mental retardation* is generally not used for the birth-to-three age group, actual incidence figures are not available. About 0.5 percent of the preschool population are identified as being mentally retarded. Learning difficulties are often not recognized, however, until the child enters school. It is therefore not surprising that this figure jumps to 10 percent in the six-to-sixteen age group.

Seventy-five percent of mental retardation is mild, 20 percent is moderate, and only 5 percent severe or profound. Mild retardation is most prevalent among lower socioeconomic groups, whereas moderate and severe mental retardation is more evenly distributed across all socioeconomic levels.

DETECTION

Possible mental retardation is suggested by delays in obtaining developmental milestones and by poor performance on formal cognitive tests. The physician, often the first professional to suspect an intellectual deficit in a very young child, is responsible for initiating referral to an appropriate assessment team.

Performance on standardized psychometric tests that is two or more standard deviations below the mean signals significant delay in cognitive function. There are, however, important cautions in interpreting the results of such tests in very young chidren:

- Tests predict better as the child gets older. They also predict better with more delayed children, since their behavior is more consistent and less variable over time. Therefore, the predictive value of standard psychometric tests is limited with very young children or children who have mild delays in cognitive development. The tests themselves are not the only reasons for caution. Allowances must be made for the significant variability in the rates of development of young children.
- Many tests are heavily related to sensorimotor function, limiting the performance of children with deficits in these areas. Children with serious chronic diseases may have temporary developmental delays due to poor nutrition, frequent hospitalizations, and lack of appropriate stimulation.
- Performance on developmental tests is to some extent dependent upon the child's experience and may therefore be limited by environmental deprivation.

New assessment techniques involving a child's ability to habituate to a stimulus and recognize a novel stimulus promise more accurate estimates of intellectual functioning, particularly when there is significant sensory and/or motor impairment.

MEDICAL MANAGEMENT

In addition to looking for the cause of mental retardation, the physician has a second important task: that of providing optimal health care, without which the mentally disabled child may not reach his or her highest potential.

Health and development are often closely intertwined, and the physician can help parents integrate the information they receive in these two areas. The physician generally has continual access to parents' perceptions and emotions. Talking to parents at frequent intervals—determining their feelings about their disabled child and providing a resource for ongoing support—is as important a role for the physician as it is for social workers, psychologists, and therapists who work with the child and family.

IMPLICATIONS FOR THE EDUCATIONAL SETTING

While the implications of mental retardation involve primarily educational and psychological development, education-related professionals can also help improve the physical health of these children by encouraging parents to arrange for a medical evaluation (if one has not already been performed) and by helping to identify ongoing health concerns which should be addressed to the child's physician.

SEE ALSO

Approach to Syndromes, Cerebral Palsy, Congenital Infections, Down Syndrome, Fetal Alcohol Syndrome, Low Birth Weight, and *Phenylketonuria and Other Metabolic Diseases*

Middle Ear Disease (Otitis Media)

James A. Blackman, M.D.

DESCRIPTION

Middle ear disease, or otitis media, is an inflammatory disease of the middle ear, common in children under six years of age. There are two types. The first, called acute otitis media, is characterized by a red, bulging, immobile eardrum, ear pain, and bacteria and pus in the middle ear. The second, called serous otitis media, is a more chronic condition of the middle ear; while it may have some of the same features as acute otitis media, the most prominent characteristic is fluid in the middle ear space, which can result in varying degrees of hearing loss.

CAUSE

The eustachian tube connects the middle ear space with the nasal cavity. It equalizes pressure between the middle ear and the atmosphere and permits drainage of secretions. Sometimes this tube does not work well or becomes blocked—most commonly by swelling of the nasal tissues, which accompanies upper respiratory infections. Fluid may then accumulate in the middle ear and allow disease-producing bacteria and viruses to cause an active infection, called acute otitis media.

In many cases, the fluid which accumulates in the middle ear during acute otitis media persists for many weeks after the infection. This accumulation of fluid and accompanying symptoms is known as serous otitis media.

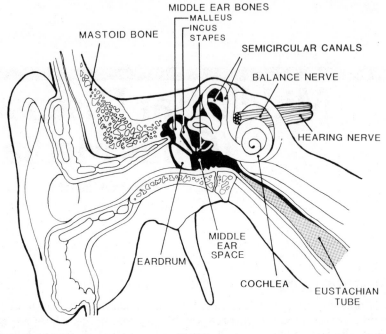

The Ear

INCIDENCE

Next to colds, otitis media is the most common reason for illness-related visits to the doctor. Ear infections are particularly common in infants and very small children; various studies have indicated that between 25 and 65 percent of children under two years of age have had at least one such infection. The incidence is higher among boys; it is also higher during cold weather months, when upper respiratory infections are common. There are, to date, no conclusive facts regarding the influence of genetic or racial factors.

DETECTION

Children with acute otitis media often complain of earache; they may rub or tug at their ears, have drainage from the ear, and occasionally show signs of hearing impairment. Examination with an otoscope will show a red, bulging eardrum. The most important clue to diagnosis is an eardrum that doesn't move well. This can be checked either with the otoscope—which can create positive or negative pressure in the ear canal—or with an electronic device called an impedance tympanometer, which can be used in an office, clinic, or school setting to provide a simple, fast, objective measure of eardrum mobility.

Otoscope

Serous otitis media, the persistence of fluid in the middle ear, is also best detected with either a pneumatic otoscope or an impedance typanometer. Initially, the eardrum may be bulging because of fluid. If this fluid is gradually absorbed, the eardrum retracts and the thick, gluelike material remaining may need to be drained surgically.

Otitis media is sometimes difficult to detect in young infants. Nonspecific symptoms—such as irritability, fever, and lethargy—should be investigated immediately. Infants and young children with colds should be watched very closely for symptoms of otitis media. So should children who have a history of ear infections and those with conditions that make them prone to ear infections (e.g., cleft palate or Down syndrome).

COURSE

Ear infections usually respond well to antibiotic treatment, but fluid in the middle ear may persist for weeks or even months following the acute infection. Children with eustachian tube dysfunction may be predisposed to recurrent infections and have difficulty eliminating fluid.

ACCOMPANYING HEALTH PROBLEMS

Recurrent otitis media, both acute and serous, can be a major problem. It puts a strain on the family and on the health care system. Even more important is that chronic, severe, and perhaps even moderate middle ear disease affects hearing and, therefore, language development and learning in general. It is still uncertain what effects mild and/or intermittent ear disease have on long-term function.

Otitis media may cause still other complications, including extension of the infection into the mastoid bone, known as mastoiditis—a condition that is difficult to treat. Another possibility is perforation of the eardrum, which, depending on the size of the hole, may or may not heal on its own. While perforation is usually not serious, it can lead to loss of function and increased susceptibility to the formation of cholesteatoma in the middle ear. Cholesteatoma is a condition in which surface cells from the external auditory canal gain entry into the middle ear space, where they begin to grow and form a tumor which can erode the incus, malleus, and stapes and invade the surrounding bones.

MEDICAL MANAGEMENT

Although some ear infections are caused by viruses—against which antibiotics are ineffective—as well as by bacteria, the usual procedure is to treat all infections with antibiotics. This is because distinguishing between the two involves the uncomfortable and costly procedure of puncturing the eardrum to obtain material for a culture (which may take days to grow). Viral infections tend to be less serious and will clear up with or without antibiotics. If bacteria are responsible and the appropriate antibiotics are administered, the infection will usually clear up in one to two weeks.

Recurrent otitis media is treated by various approaches, including (1) low doses of prophylactic antibiotics, especially during seasons of highest incidence; (2) antihistamines and decongestants; and (3) surgical placement of tubes in the eardrum to allow continuous drainage and provide an alternate route for ventilation of the middle ear space. No one procedure is unequivocally preferred; all three have benefits and liabilities. While antibiotics are generally effective, bacteria tend to develop a resistance to those which are administered repeatedly. Furthermore, unless the antibiotics are taken as prescribed—and often they are not—they are likely to be ineffective.

While various decongestants are commonly used for prevention and treatment, their effectiveness has never been scientifically proven. Presumably, they shrink the swollen membranes of the nose, enabling the eustachian tube to remain open and function properly.

Surgical drainage of the middle ear (myringotomy) and insertion of tubes into the eardrum are also controversial. Although there is as yet no uncontestable research to support their effectiveness, these procedures—when appropriate—appear to improve the function of the middle ear and decrease the number of infections.

The most prudent course at the present time is to treat acute infections with appropriate antibiotics, to follow the status of the middle ear with pneumatic otoscopy or impedance tympanometry, and to consider various treatments for recurrent acute infections and persistent serous fluid in the middle ear.

IMPLICATIONS FOR EDUCATION

Because of the age group served and the types of disabilities encountered, ear infections are very common in children participating in early education and therapeutic programs. It is therefore very important for teachers and therapists to understand the nature of otitis media and to appreciate the impact it has on health and developmental function. Acute infections result in absences as well as in general irritability, either of which may reduce the effectiveness of the educational program.

By noting changes in the behavior of children at high risk for ear infections, education-related professials can help identify the child with possible ear disease; by watching for signs of improvement (often educational programs have impedance typanometers), they can aid in proper medical management. Such information is valuable in determining the most appropriate timing and type of therapy for persistent serous otitis media. Health care providers and early intervention staff should work closely together when dealing with diseases of the middle ear.

SEE ALSO

Cleft Palate, Down Syndrome, and *Hearing Impairment*

Myelomeningocele

Mark L. Wolraich, M.D.

DESCRIPTION

Myelomeningocele, also known as meningomyelocele and spina bifida, is a midline defect of the skin, spinal column, and spinal cord.

During the latter part of the first month of pregnancy, when the child is developing in the uterus, the spinal cord (myelo-) and vertebrae around it do not form properly. In the normal child, the spinal cord forms into a straight column, covered first by membranes (meningo-) and then by a bony spine. In the child with myelomeningocele, the membranes pouch out at some point along the back. As the spinal cord develops, it does not follow a straight column but pushes out instead into the membranous sac (-cele), where it does not form in the normal way. Some or all of the nerves coming out of the spine below the sac are not hooked up properly to the spinal cord and thus to the brain.

SPINAL CORD

VERTEBRAE

VERTEBRA (Bone)

MENINGES

SPINAL CORD

Normal Spine   Myelomeningocele

There are two other types of open spine defect: meningocele and spina bifida occulta. With meningocele, the spinal cord itself does not pouch out, only the membranes surrounding it. With spina bifida occulta, the back of the vertebrae fail to form, but there are no abnormalities in the membranes, spinal cord, or skin.

Children with myelomeningocele may be characterized by hydrocephalus, mental retardation, and, depending upon the location of the defect along the spinal column, lack of control of leg muscles, lack of bladder and bowel control, lack of sensation in the skin, and/or curvature of the spine (scoliosis).

CAUSE

The exact cause of myelomeningocele is not known; it may, in fact, result from a combination of causes. There is no proven link between this condition and any medication, infection, or environmental condition. Nor are parents carriers of a gene that specifically causes myelomeningocele, though they may carry genes which make them susceptible to various nongenetic (e.g., environmental) factors known to be associated with it.

INCIDENCE

Myelomeningocele is one of the most common developmental defects of the nervous system; the incidence is about one in every thousand births. The chance of having a second child with this condition is somewhere between 1 in 20 and 1 in 40.

DETECTION

Prenatal

Myelomeningocele may be detected in the fetus through amniocentesis—by measuring the amount of alpha fetal protein (AFP) and acetylcholinesterase in the amniotic fluid. These proteins are found in high concentration in spinal fluid, which, in the child with myelomeningocele, leaks through the membrane and into the amniotic fluid surrounding the fetus.

Another, easier method of testing for myelomeningocele in the fetus is measuring the amount of alpha fetal protein in the mother's blood. This test, which must be done between the twelfth and fourteenth weeks of gestation, is not as accurate as amniocentesis, for which it is sometimes used as a preliminary.

Sometimes sound waves bounced off the fetus (ultrasonography) make the defect visible. This procedure is not always reliable, however.

Postnatal

Initial diagnosis is not difficult because the spinal lesion is present at birth and easily observed. The extent of the problem can be determined by assessing the lesion itself as well as the muscle groups affected. In rare cases, the defect is covered by skin and goes undetected in the newborn period.

COURSE

Myelomeningocele is a static condition; that is, there is no progression of the defect. However, secondary problems (urinary, for example) can worsen and require intensive management.

ACCOMPANYING HEALTH PROBLEMS

Hydrocephalus

In about 80 percent of children with myelomeningocele, the spinal fluid is prevented from leaving the brain and being absorbed into the blood stream. The resultant increase in pressure may cause brain damage and, hence, mental retardation.

Muscle control

Because the nerves to the lower part of the body are not properly connected to the spinal cord and brain, there may be little or no control of leg muscles. The higher up the defect is on the spinal cord, the greater the paralysis. Most myelomeningocele defects occur in the thoracic, lumbar, or sacral regions of the spine:

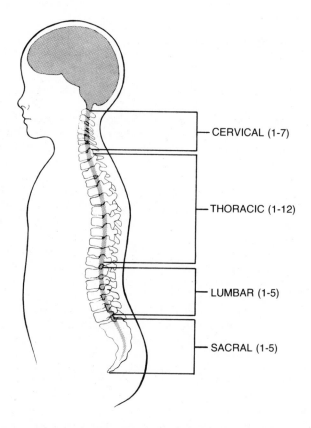

CERVICAL (1-7)

THORACIC (1-12)

LUMBAR (1-5)

SACRAL (1-5)

Regions of the Spine

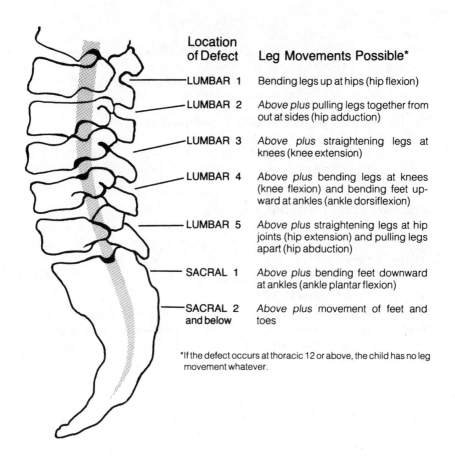

Location of Defect	Leg Movements Possible*
LUMBAR 1	Bending legs up at hips (hip flexion)
LUMBAR 2	*Above plus* pulling legs together from out at sides (hip adduction)
LUMBAR 3	*Above plus* straightening legs at knees (knee extension)
LUMBAR 4	*Above plus* bending legs at knees (knee flexion) and bending feet upward at ankles (ankle dorsiflexion)
LUMBAR 5	*Above plus* straightening legs at hip joints (hip extension) and pulling legs apart (hip abduction)
SACRAL 1	*Above plus* bending feet downward at ankles (ankle plantar flexion)
SACRAL 2 and below	*Above plus* movement of feet and toes

*If the defect occurs at thoracic 12 or above, the child has no leg movement whatever.

Relationship Between Level of Defect and Leg Movement—*Incomplete lesions account for variations among children with myelomeningocele.*

Problems with bladder and bowel control

Because the nerves involved in bladder control come from the lower part of the spinal cord (the second, third, and fourth sacral segments), most children with myelomeningocele have neurogenic bladders. This means they may not feel the urge to urinate or have control of the urinary sphincter. A neurogenic bladder, if not cared for properly, may cause damage to the kidneys, either because the urine cannot get out properly (causing pressure on the kidneys) or because not all the urine is emptied from the bladder (causing infections). Treatments are available to prevent urinary tract infection and subsequent kidney damage.

The nerves involved in bowel control also come from the lower part of the spinal cord, and children with myelomeningocele frequently have neurogenic bowels. This may result in constipation and bowel movement accidents (incontinence).

Curvature of the spine (scoliosis)

Due to poor muscle control and the structural defect of the spine, straight alignment is sometimes not maintained. This can lead to a fixed tilt of the pelvis and curvature of the spine, causing poor sitting balance and excessive pressure on certain areas of the skin.

Problems with psychosocial development

Both the nature of the defect and the functional difficulties which accompany it may place strains on parent-child relationships. As the child grows older, functional limitations may lead to psychological and social maladjustment.

Pressure sores (decubitus ulcers)

Many children with myelomeningocele lack sensation in their lower extremities, making them prone to pressure sores. The skin should be checked frequently for reddened areas—the first sign of a problem.

MEDICAL MANAGEMENT

The complexity of the dysfunction and the number of organ systems involved demand the participation of many surgical and medical specialists and health-related personnel. An interdisciplinary team is frequently necessary to provide appropriate coordinated care.

Spinal lesion

To prevent germs from entering the open defect and causing serious infections in the spinal cord and brain, the lesion is generally repaired surgically within the first 24 to 48 hours of life.

Hydrocephalus

To prevent damage to brain tissue, the increased intracranial pressure is treated with a shunt, which is surgically placed, usually within the first two months of life.

Urinary tract

Urologic management begins at birth. In the past, various surgical procedures were used to redirect urinary flow and preserve kidney function. But conservative therapies now appear to be effective. These include periodic assessment of urinary tract function and intermittent catheterization to help prevent both urinary tract infections and "accidents."

Orthopedics

Evaluation begins at birth. The aims of management procedures are to preserve normal joint structures, to release contractures, to correct deformities, and to facilitate weight bearing and, where possible, ambulation. (Many of these children can learn to walk with the aid of braces and crutches.)

Psychosocial problems

Support for both child and family must begin with the child's birth and continue throughout his lifetime.

IMPLICATIONS FOR EDUCATION

The constant occurrence of acute problems—such as shunt malfunction, urinary tract infection, and repeated hospitalizations and surgery—combines with the socially limiting nature of such problems to affect almost every aspect of the child's performance in an educational setting.

Myelomeningocele generally has no effect on a child's stamina, although the accompanying hydrocephalus may cause attention disorders, learning disorders, and even mental retardation. Educational assessments are necessary to determine what types of learning problems—if any—a child may have.

Because of the damaged nerves along the spine, children with myelomeningocele may not experience the amount of weight bearing necessary for bone development and strengthening; they are therefore more prone to fractures in the lower extremities. Too, they may lack sensation in certain areas of the skin, increasing considerably the risk of burns, abrasions, and pressure ulcers. They may also lack bladder or bowel control and be participating in special bladder and bowel regimes at school. Because these children are less active than normal children, they are prone to obesity and may be following certain nutrition recommendations. Too, the excess weight can impede ambulation and contribute to the development of pressure sores.

The extent of physical and mental problems varies with the location of the defect; some children with myelomeningocele have relatively few of the problems listed here.

SEE ALSO

Bracing, Defects in Brain Development, Hydrocephalus, and *Mental Retardation*

Neuroanatomy

James A. Blackman, M.D.

The Nervous System

THE CENTRAL NERVOUS SYSTEM (CNS)

BRAIN—Includes the cerebrum, cerebellum, midbrain, pons, and medulla oblongata.

SPINAL CORD—Divided into cervical (neck), thoracic (chest), lumbar (lower back), and sacral (lowest back) sections.

THE PERIPHERAL NERVOUS SYSTEM (PNS)

These nerves connect with the brain or spinal cord but originate or terminate outside these structures in areas such as the skin and muscle.

MOTOR NERVES—Innervate the skeletal muscles, such as the biceps of the arm.

SENSORY NERVES—Transmit impulses from receptors for pain, taste, muscle tension, touch, and other stimuli.

AUTONOMIC NERVES—Innervate cardiac muscle, glands, the muscles of the intestines, and other organs not under voluntary control.

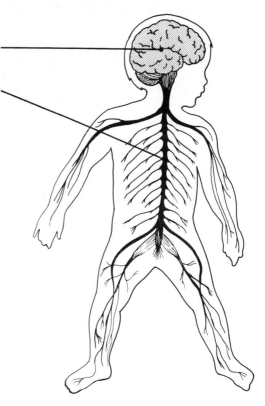

The Central and Peripheral Nervous Systems

Areas of Specialized Function

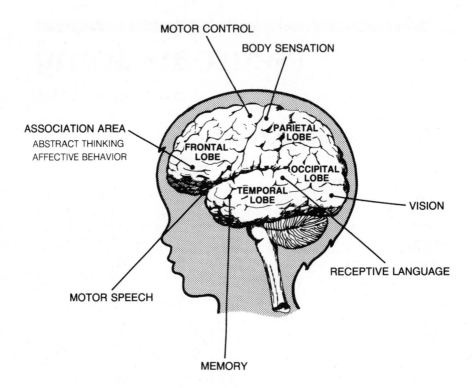

Topography of the Cerebral Cortex

Important Structures of the Brain and Their Functions

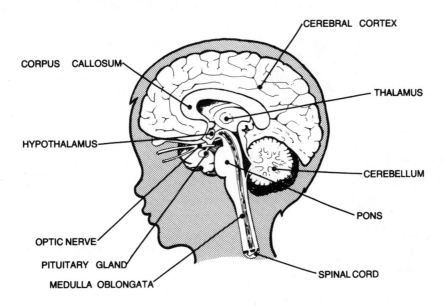

CEREBELLUM—The part of the brain responsible for muscle synergy and coordination.

CEREBRAL CORTEX—The surface gray matter of the brain, generally considered responsible for "thinking" and volitional activity.

CORPUS CALLOSUM—Joins the cerebral hemispheres, allowing them to "communicate" with each other.

HYPOTHALAMUS—Regulates the autonomic nervous system, causing sweating, changes in heart rate, and intestinal contractions; also regulates appetite, body temperature, and the physical expressions of emotion (e.g., flushing of the skin).

MEDULLA OBLONGATA—Nerve fibers from higher brain centers pass through here on their way to the spinal cord. The hearing and balance nerves enter the brain here. Certain nerves which control and receive information from the mouth, throat, neck, heart, and abdominal viscera leave and enter here. Also, nerve fibers from the motor strip of each cerebral hemisphere cross over here to control movement on the opposite side of the body.

OPTIC NERVE—The route traveled by visual impulses.

PITUITARY GLAND—Releases hormones regulating water balance in the body, ovulation, growth, thyroid gland function, and the release of other hormones by the adrenal gland.

PONS—Nerves to and from the face originate and terminate here.

SPINAL CORD—Conduit for motor and sensory fibers going to and from the brain.

THALAMUS—The switching station for impulses going to the cerebral cortex.

Midline Section of the Brain

Control of Voluntary Movement

(1) A command from the association areas of the brain stimulates the motor area of the **FRONTAL LOBE,** triggering impulses.

(2) The impulses travel down a nerve "tract," or bundle, which converges with other nerve fibers from the motor area to form the **CORTICOSPINAL (PYRAMIDAL) TRACT.**

(3) At the lowest level of the **MEDULLA,** the fibers of the corticospinal tract cross over to the opposite side, then travel down the spinal cord.

(4) The corticospinal tract connects with a **PERIPHERAL NERVE;** this leaves the spinal cord and

(5) carries the impulses to the **MUSCLE,** causing it to contract and make the desired movement.

Control of Voluntary Movement

Refinement and coordination of movement is dependent on input from several other important structures outside the pyramidal system. The basal ganglia modulate pyramidal tract activity, and the cerebellum coordinates muscles so that they perform smoothly and accurately. The vestibular system of the inner ear helps the body maintain equilibrium; and special sensory organs in the skin, eyes, muscles, tendons, and joints provide the brain with continuous feedback regarding the position and movement of the limbs.

Damage in any of these areas can interfere with the execution of voluntary movement:

Damaged area	Result of damage
• Corticospinal tract or motor areas of the cerebral cortex	• Spasticity with some paralysis
• Basal ganglia	• Movement disorders
• Cerebellum	• Problems with balance and coordination (ataxia)
• Peripheral nerve and muscle	• Weakness or flaccidity

The Anatomy of a Deep Tendon Reflex (DTR)—The Knee Jerk

When a muscle or tendon is suddenly stretched by a reflex hammer . . .

(1) **SENSORY FIBERS** in the muscle detect the sudden change in muscle length and

(2) send an impulse to the spinal cord along a **SENSORY NERVE,**

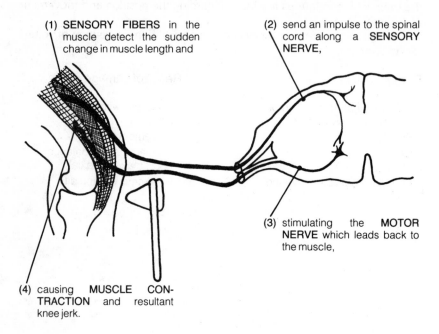

(3) stimulating the **MOTOR NERVE** which leads back to the muscle,

(4) causing **MUSCLE CONTRACTION** and resultant knee jerk.

The Knee Jerk

This same reflex response can be elicited in any skeletal muscle by rapid stretching. Although this reflex involves a circuit that is independent of the brain, input from the brain is what keeps it in check. If the brain is unable to control this response (as might be the case, for example, when there is damage to the corticospinal tract), it would be increased. That is, the knee jerk would be exaggerated. This is typically seen in the spastic type of cerebral palsy. Disruption of the circuit itself—usually in the spinal cord, along the peripheral motor nerve, or in the muscle—may, conversely, result in a dampened response or no response at all. Exaggerated or reduced responses during the neurological examination may help pinpoint trouble sites.

The Neurological Examination

David P. Schor, M.D.

An essential part of the evaluation of any child with a developmental disability is the neurological examination. This assessment—along with a history of the child's health and development, findings from other parts of the physical examination, and the results of laboratory tests—provides clues to diagnosis and proper treatment.

MEDICAL HISTORY

Before actually examining the infant, the physician usually collects information about the child's problem—when it was first noticed, whether it has been improving or getting worse, and whether there are any health concerns, such as recurrent ear infections or episodes of vomiting or diarrhea. Information is also sought regarding the family and previous life events which may be linked to the child's current difficulties. Parents or caretakers are questioned about **(1)** diseases that run in the family; **(2)** problems the mother may have had during pregnancy, labor, or delivery; **(3)** unusual behavior or poor health of the child after birth; **(4)** delay or deviation in development; and **(5)** possible environmental stresses. Finally, a systematic review of each organ system yields information about hearing and vision, heart and lung function, the skeleton, and so forth.

PHYSICAL EXAMINATION

General observations

With infants and young children, simple observation may be as revealing (or more so) than the actual hands-on assessment. Hence, the neurological examination begins there. Does the child appear well? Adequately nourished? Of normal body proportions? Is the level of alertness or responsiveness to stimuli significantly heightened? Diminished?

How much and how well the child moves may indicate whether there is damage to the nervous system and, if so, to what part; for instance, if the arm and leg on the left side appear floppy or stiff, there may be damage to the right side of the brain (which controls movement on the left side of the body).

The head

Abnormal head size or shape is often associated with abnormal growth and development of the brain. This is especially likely if there is delay in the child's development or if the unusual size or shape is not found among normal family members. Small head size (microcephaly) may be due to defects in brain development, intrauterine infections, postnatal mishaps (such as birth asphyxia), or certain metabolic disorders. An abnormally large head size (macrocephaly), unless it is a familial variation, is usually due to an accumulation of fluid in and around the brain (hydrocephalus). The cause for excessive brain growth (megalencephaly), a rare condition often accompanied by mental retardation, is unknown.

The eyes

Examination of the eye and its movements can provide clues to neurologic abnormalities. Unequal eye movements, failure of the pupils to react to light, or rapid, involuntary jerking of the eyes (nystagmus) may be caused by disturbances in the visual pathways or by problems with eye muscle control.

Eye movements can be assessed by observing the infant's reactions to a moving, striped pattern or by having the child track a small, interesting object. Pupil reactions are checked by shining bright lights first in one eye and then in the other. Using small magnifying lenses combined with a light source (ophthalmoscope), the physician can also directly inspect the retina and the optic nerve at the back of each eye. This inspection may reveal signs of (1) pressure in the brain from a tumor or accumulation of fluid, (2) diseases with manifestations in the eye (e.g., toxoplasmosis), or (3) rare genetic conditions (e.g., Tay-Sachs disease).

The ears

Infants are screened for major problems in hearing by observing their responses to vocalizations or other noises (e.g., a rattle or bell). In addition, the eardrum and middle ear are examined with an otoscope. The child with suspected hearing problems should be referred to an audiologist for formal testing.

Significant hearing impairment usually results from a buildup of fluid in the middle ear. At times, however, it is a result of abnormalities—some of them inherited—in the nerves which transform sound into impulses and then transmit those impulses to the brain.

Nerves of the head and neck

Specialized nerve fibers called cranial nerves control specific face and head movements; they also transmit information about sensory stimuli which reach the head. Abnormalities along these pathways may be detected by observing for asymmetry in facial expressions and in movements of the tongue and palate.

Muscle function

In addition to observing the infant or young child's voluntary activities, the examiner assesses both muscle tone and strength. Muscle tone is the amount of resistance the examiner feels in response to passive movement—to having the arm moved back and forth by the examiner, for example. Stiffness (hypertonia) or floppiness (hypotonia) is often seen with damage to those areas of the brain and spinal cord which control motor activity. Floppiness may also result from abnormalities in the nerves leading from the spinal column to the muscles or from abnormalities in the muscles themselves. The examiner checks tone and strength by observing the child's movements and by passively moving the child's head and extremities through their full range of motion.

Reflexes

Reflexes are predictable movements in response to various stimuli. For example, an infant of less than three months will usually grasp a finger that is placed firmly in the palm of its hand; or a newborn whose cheek is stroked will usually turn to face that side (this is known as "rooting") and make sucking movements. Other neonatal reflexes involve the infant's whole body. For instance, the child reacts to a sudden noise or change of position by extending the arms and legs briefly, then bringing them back together as though to hug a nearby object (the Moro response).

Many reflexes which are present in the neonatal period normally disappear with time. Their persistence beyond the time of anticipated decline may signal brain abnormalities. As the infant grows older, most neonatal reflexes are replaced by new automatic responses (e.g., righting and equilibrium), which can be elicited during examinations. These are prerequisites for new skills, such as sitting, crawling, and walking. The appearance of new responses is often delayed, however, if the earlier, "primitive" reflexes continue.

Deep tendon reflexes are important indicators of the function of the neurological system. One such reflex is the knee jerk. A heightened response—an excessive knee jerk—suggests the possibility of damage to the brain itself or to the nerve that travels along the spinal cord from the motor cortex of the brain (the corticospinal tract). A poor or negative response suggests one of three things: problems with the nerve running from the spinal cord to the muscle, problems with the muscle itself, or general central nervous system depression.

Another sign of central nervous system dysfunction is an abnormal Babinski response. When the bottom of the foot is stroked, the toes should bend downward. If the toes bend upward and fan out, the response is considered abnormal.

Yet another response which suggests problems in the central nervous system—particularly in the motor cortex or in the corticospinal tract—is clonus. Clonus is repeated muscle jerking which occurs when the muscle is suddenly stretched (as happens, for instance, when the foot is bent upward).

Other findings

Findings in other organ systems may suggest nervous system dysfunction. For example, children with neurofibromatosis, a disease which affects the skin as well as the nervous system, generally develop areas of increased pigmentation on the skin (*café au lait* spots), which may suggest the diagnosis of this disease before neurological symptoms are evident.

Another rare condition with important neurological manifestations is the Sturge-Weber syndrome. Abnormal growth of blood vessels in early fetal life produces a purplish, nonelevated area of the skin, commonly on one side of the face. Similar blood vessel abnormalities may also occur in the brain covering (meninges) below the affected facial skin, producing faulty brain growth and development, with resultant seizures, mental retardation, and motor disability.

Abnormal findings in the physical examination or a history of delayed developmental milestones (particularly in the motor area) during early infancy must be viewed in light of an objective measure of the child's general developmental level. A general developmental screening test is done to determine if there is need for a more complete, interdisciplinary evaluation.

Depending on what has been learned from the patient history and physical exam, selected laboratory studies may help pinpoint the trouble. The most commonly employed tests include blood analyses, X-rays, computerized axial tomography (CAT) scans, and electroencephalograms (EEGs). The physician generally tries to gain the most information with the fewest tests and the least discomfort to the child.

INTERPRETATION

The greatest skill of the examiner lies in interpreting and integrating the information obtained from all of the above techniques. All physicians are trained to perform a neurological assessment and to interpret the findings; with difficult cases, however, it may be necessary to rely on the expertise of a specialist in this field—the pediatric neurologist.

SEE ALSO

Cerebral Palsy, Computerized Axial Tomography, Defects in Brain Development, Electroencephalography, The Floppy Infant, and *Neuroanatomy*

Orthopedic Problems

James A. Blackman, M.D.

Infants may be born with or acquire problems with bones, joints, and muscles. This chapter will describe some of the more common orthopedic disorders of the foot, knee, hip, spine, and other areas of the body.

THE FOOT

Metatarsus adductus

The forefoot turns inward but the ankle and heel are in their normal positions, a problem which may be related to the compression of the fetus in the uterus. Mild and flexible cases are treated with stretching exercises; rigid deformities may require casting in early infancy. Generally, the longer treatment is delayed, the more difficult it is to remold the foot into a normal position.

Metatarsus Adductus

Club foot (talipes equino-cavovarus)

With this condition, certain muscles are shortened, and the tissues surrounding the joints are fixed, causing the foot to turn inward and upward. Treatment, which includes passive correction and prolonged casting, should begin as soon after birth as possible.

Club Foot

Calcaneovalgus

The bones of the foot are usually in normal alignment, but the foot is turned outward, the ankle upward. This deformity is flexible; if treated soon after birth by daily passive stretching of the soft tissue, it may improve spontaneously.

Flat feet *(pes planus)*

Babies' feet tend to look flat because of a thick layer of fat tissue on the bottoms. With time, this layer disappears and the arch usually becomes evident. In the otherwise normal child, treatment for flat feet is necessary only rarely—corrective surgery almost never. Children beyond the age of three who experience discomfort may use arch supports to distribute weight evenly.

Flat Feet

Toeing in

Toeing in—that is, turning inward of one or both of the lower extremities—is caused by a condition or combination of conditions involving the foot, the larger bone between the knee and ankle (tibia), and/or the bone between the hip and knee (femur). Toeing in is commonly caused by metatarsus adductus (discussed above). If the child has a flexible foot, it usually corrects itself; otherwise, cast treatment may be necessary. A twisting inward of the tibia (tibial torsion) can cause severe or persistent turning in of the entire foot; this is commonly treated by night splints, although there is some disagreement about their effectiveness. A third cause of toeing in is a turning inward of the femur (femoral anteversion). Present in all babies, this generally corrects itself with age and is helped little by shoe corrections. Even in persistent cases, no treatment is necessary except encouraging long- or crossed-leg sitting rather than W-sitting.

Toeing In

Toeing out

Toeing out is normal when children begin to walk, and in most cases correction is spontaneous. If, however, toeing out persists after a period of independent walking, orthopedic consultation is recommended; the condition may be due to a twisting outward of the large bone between the knee and ankle (external tibial torsion) or it may be caused by flat feet.

Congenital rocker-bottom foot (vertical talus)

Congenital malposition of the bones of the foot results in a characteristic rocker-bottom shape to the underside of the foot, a problem which requires orthopedic consultation.

THE KNEE

Knock knees *(genu valgum)* **and bow legs** *(genu varum)*

These problems generally do not require treatment, although at times wedges (lifts) in the shoes are prescribed. Mild bowing of the lower extremities is typical in the infant and very young child and usually corrects itself spontaneously by 18 months to two years. If not, the physician will search for specific causes, such as abnormal muscle tone, nutritional deficiencies (rickets), abnormal bone growth, or other diseases.

Knock Knees   Bow Legs

Abnormal hyperextensibility of the knees joint *(genu recurvatum)*

Normally, straightening of the knee stops when the bones of the upper and lower leg are in alignment. Lax joint support tissues (as found in Ehlers-Danlos syndrome) or abnormal muscle tone (spastic diplegia) may cause children to stand with their knees hyperextended. In severe cases bracing may be necessary.

THE HIP

Congenital dislocation of the hip (CDH)

This problem results from abnormal development of some of the components of the hip joint. At times, the head of the thigh bone (femur) may be totally out of the hip socket, or the supporting tissue may be lax and allow this bone to move in and out of the socket when manipulated by a doctor. The cause of this problem, which affects females more often than males, is not known, though it is very likely that a number of factors is involved, including breech delivery, hormonal changes in the mother during late pregnancy, and positioning of hip after birth (CDH occurs more frequently in some culture groups which swaddle their infants or wrap them to cradle boards).

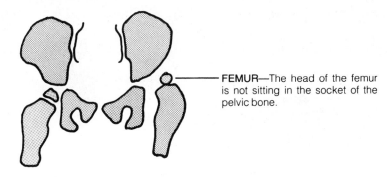

FEMUR—The head of the femur is not sitting in the socket of the pelvic bone.

Congenital Dislocation of the Hip

Children are checked for CDH during the regular physical examination in the newborn period and repeatedly during the first year of life. The examiner attempts to gently move the femoral head in and out of the hip socket. Normally this is not possible. X-rays are not useful in the newborn period but may help to confirm the diagnosis in older infants. Children with spina bifida and certain types of cerebral palsy are prone to dislocation of the hip at any age and are therefore monitored closely for this problem.

The goal of treatment is to return the femoral head to its normal position within the hip socket (acetabulum). To prevent joint inflammation (arthritis), treatment should begin as soon as possible. Newborns are treated with splints, older babies with casting or surgery.

THE SPINE

Infantile scoliosis

Many times, curvature of the spine (scoliosis) in children ages birth to three is idiopathic; that is, the cause is unknown. This condition—which is very rare in the United States—is more common among boys and children with low birth weight and muscle disorders. In about 85 percent of cases, idiopathic scoliosis disappears on its own, but in the remaining 15 percent, the curve may worsen and lead to severe deformity.

Congenital scoliosis

Another type of scoliosis is caused by abnormal development of the bony parts of the spine (vertebrae). Children born with this type (which is confirmed by X-rays) need close follow-up; if the defect is progressive, they may require surgery.

INFANTILE SCOLIOSIS

CONGENITAL SCOLIOSIS

Comparison of Infantile and Congenital Scoliosis—*With infantile scoliosis, the bony parts of the spine are normally developed; with congenital scoliosis, they are malformed.*

Neuromuscular scoliosis

A third type of scoliosis occurs as a result of neuromuscular disease. With cerebral palsy, for example, the degree of muscle tone may be greater on one side than on the other, causing unequal forces on the spine. This and other conditions which are characterized by abnormal muscle tone allow the child to sit or stand with the spine out of alignment, resulting in curvature. With neuromuscular scoliosis, attention should be given to the underlying disease. Treatment includes proper positioning, bracing, and, occasionally, surgery.

THE JOINTS

Anthrogryposis

Babies are sometimes born with various joints compressed and positioned at abnormal angles (anthrogryposis). This congenital deformity is caused by neuromuscular problems in the fetus, too little amniotic fluid, or structural abnormalities of the uterus—all of which inhibit the fetus from moving in the uterus.

Anthrogryposis multiplex congenita is a severe form of this disorder characterized by many involved joints as well as by other types of bony and muscular abnormalities.

Mild cases of both these conditions are treated by passive exercises; more severe cases may require gradual correction of deformities by splints, casts, or surgery.

SEE ALSO

Bracing, Cerebral Palsy, Myelomeningocele, and *Positioning*

Perinatal Injury

James A. Blackman, M.D.

Jason B. was a 4,200-gram, full-term infant, born to a gravida III, para II, abortus I, 29-year-old woman. The pregnancy was complicated by preeclampsia and gestational diabetes. Labor was induced because of maternal high blood pressure. The amniotic sac was artificially ruptured, and the fluid contained thick meconium. Monitoring indicated fetal distress, and so delivery was by emergency cesarean section. Apgars were 1 at one minute and 5 at five minutes. Jason required vigorous resuscitation. Problems in the early newborn period included aspiration pneumonia, hypoxia, hypoglycemia, and jaundice. Seizures appeared on the second day of life. He had continuing feeding problems and was hypotonic at the time of discharge.

This is a typical, though abbreviated, case history of a difficult perinatal period which will have a profound impact on the child's future growth and development. This report and others like it contain certain terms commonly used by medical professionals, many of which are defined in this chapter. (The information presented here is not all-inclusive; some of the terms may be found in other, relevant sections of this manual.)

TERMS APPLIED TO A WOMAN TO SIGNIFY HER PREGNANCY AND BIRTHING HISTORY

Gravida
Latin for pregnant woman; she is called *gravida* I during the first pregnancy, *gravida* II during the second, etc.

Para
Also Latin, meaning a woman who has borne a live child. A *para* II is a woman who has borne two live children, etc.

Abortus

A miscarriage or delivery of a fetus with no chance of survival.

Stillborn

The child, though mature enough to survive outside the uterus, is born dead.

MATERNAL CONDITIONS WHICH AFFECT THE GROWING FETUS

Prenatal care

Studies have shown a higher incidence of prematurity and complications in newborns whose mothers did not receive adequate medical supervision. Contact with a physician early in the pregnancy facilitates the detection of conditions which may adversely affect the fetus and newborn child; it also allows treatment which may ameliorate, if not prevent, complications.

Maternal disease

All acute and chronic diseases are potentially harmful to the fetus. Asthma, seizure disorders, and hypertension in the mother are a few of the diseases whose inadequate treatment may produce adverse effects. Careful monitoring of these diseases during pregnancy is essential to fetal well-being.

Rh disease

A woman with Rh negative blood may have an infant with Rh positive blood. If minute amounts of blood from the infant enter the mother's circulation—which usually happens at the time of delivery—they are recognized as foreign by the mother's system; her body reacts by developing an immunity to that type of blood. Antibodies against Rh positive blood remain in the mother's circulatory system and, in subsequent pregnancies, pass through the placenta to the fetus. Unless the unborn child has Rh negative blood like the mother, these antibodies will destroy the child's red blood cells, causing severe anemia. A mother with Rh negative blood should be given a special injection immediately after the first and each subsequent delivery to blunt her antibody responses to Rh positive blood cells from the baby, thereby preventing Rh disease with subsequent pregnancies.

Diabetes mellitus

Part of the routine testing for a newly pregnant woman is a urine check for sugar. This is because women with diabetes must have their blood sugars carefully controlled during pregnancy to insure proper growth of the fetus. Certain women who show no signs of diabetes prior to pregnancy may do so during pregnancy. A special diet and, at times, insulin may be necessary to control blood sugar.

Toxemia

Toxemia of pregnancy, the cause of which is unknown, appears to affect the kidneys, resulting in varying degrees of high blood pressure, protein in the urine, and fluid retention. Most likely to be affected are young women during their early pregnancies. Management consists of careful observation, control of blood pressure, and, in the case of uncontrollable high blood pressure or seizures, prompt delivery to save both the baby and the mother. The early, milder stage of this disease is sometimes called preeclampsia, eclampsia being the later, severe form, which is characterized by grand mal seizures. High blood pressure, a symptom of toxemia in the mother, can result in poor fetal growth as well as separation of the placenta from the uterine wall with resultant hemorrhage *(abruptio placentae)*.

Teratogens

There are many agents in the environment—some recognized, others not—which may injure the fetus. Among these, in all probability, are environmental pollutants over which the pregnant woman has no control. Agents which are known to have adverse effects, however, can and should be avoided. Among these are certain drugs, alcohol, cigarettes, and unnecessary irradiation.

CONDITIONS AND TERMS WHICH APPLY TO THE INFANT DURING LABOR, DELIVERY, OR THE EARLY NEWBORN PERIOD

Fetal monitoring

Recent techniques make it possible to monitor the heart rate of the infant during labor. An electrode may be attached externally (to the mother's abdomen) or internally (directly to the baby's scalp) to observe the infant's response to uterine contractions and to detect early signs of fetal distress. Another electrode is generally used (either internally or externally) to monitor the length and intensity of the intrauterine contractions.

Cesarean section

Cesarean section (C-section) is the delivery of the fetus through incisions in the abdominal and uterine walls. The indications for a C-section are **(1)** inability of the fetus to pass through the pelvic outlet of the mother, **(2)** prolonged labor, **(3)** *placenta previa*, in which the placenta overlies the opening of the uterus, **(4)** severe toxemia, and **(5)** fetal distress. Other situations—including a previous cesarean section or breech (other than head first) presentation—may also be viewed as cause for a C-section, depending on the doctor and/or local custom.

Apgars

Apgars are scores given to a newborn infant by a nurse or physician, usually at one and five minutes following delivery. They are a useful means of communicating the newborn's general status and adaptation to extrauterine life. The maximum Apgar score in ten.

CRITERIA FOR APGAR SCORES

	0	1	2
Color	Blue-pale	Extremities blue, rest of body pink	Completely pink
Heart rate	Absent	Below 100	Over 100
Respiratory effort	Absent	Weak, irregular	Good, crying
Muscle tone	Limp	Some flexion of extremities	Active motion
Reflex irritability (catheter in nostril)	None	Grimace	Cough/ sneeze

Efforts have been made to correlate Apgar scores with future developmental and neurological states. While very low scores do not invariably lead to significant future problems, they do indicate significant distress during labor and delivery and warrant close observation of the infant.

Resuscitation

Low or absent heart and/or breathing rates require immediate measures to stimulate or mechanically provide circulation and respiration. Delays in instituting such procedures may result in permanent neurological damage.

Asphyxia

Failure to begin breathing after delivery is a major manifestation of asphyxia, a condition characterized by too little oxygen in the blood, elevated levels of carbon dioxide in the blood and tissues, and disturbance of the acid-base balance. Circumstances which may lead to asphyxia include **(1)** compression of the umbilical cord, **(2)** premature separation of the placenta, **(3)** sustained contraction of the uterus, **(4)** an umbilical cord that is wrapped tightly around the neck or body, **(5)** damage to the head and brain during the birth process, and **(6)** depression of the infant's breathing caused by drugs administered to the mother during the late stages of labor. The longer the baby has gone without sufficient oxygen, the longer it will take for him to respond to resuscitation. Thus, the quicker the response, the better the chances for a fast and full recovery.

Meconium

Meconium is a thick, sticky brown substance which is normally passed in a bowel movement during the first few days of life. Passage of this material before delivery is one sign of fetal distress (insufficient oxygen, for example, may cause various negative reactions in the child, including the passage of meconium). Furthermore, the meconium may get inside the mouth as the child moves through the birth canal, then enter the trachea and lungs with the first breath. Meconium is highly irritating and can cause severe inflammation of the lungs (pneumonitis). When this substance cannot be removed from the baby's mouth prior to the first breath, it must be sucked out of the upper air passageway (trachea) as quickly as possible.

Jaundice

Jaundice is a yellowish color of the skin and whites of the eyes caused by an accumulation of bilirubin, a by-product of the breakdown of red blood cells. Normally, bilirubin is picked up by the liver and passed into the intestine through the bile ducts of the liver and gallbladder. The liver in the newborn, however, is slow in removing this substance from the blood. Moreover, the trauma of the birth process may bring about an increase in the breakdown of red blood cells.

While mild jaundice requires no treatment, there are instances in which it may be necessary to reduce the amount of bilirubin in the blood. For example, Rh disease and other maternal-infant blood incompatibilities may cause the red cells to break down at a rate far exceeding the liver's ability to remove the bilirubin; also, in some infants, especially those who are preterm, the liver may not be able to remove this substance efficiently. Excess bilirubin is therefore quite common in newborns and not usually cause for concern. Very high levels, however, are known to cause damage to the brain (kernicterus) and resultant cerebral palsy. There are two common treatments: when the degree of elevation is moderate, special-wavelength fluorescent lights are used to break down the bilirubin in the skin; in more severe cases, it is necessary to exchange the baby's blood with donor blood.

Sepsis/meningitis

Newborns, particularly preterm babies, have a lowered resistance to infection, making them susceptible to various bacterial, fungal, and viral organisms. The insertion of tubes (e.g., for intravenous feeding) provides an avenue of entry for infectious organisms. Since infection of the blood, spinal cord, and brain can have a devastating effect on the baby, most infants in intensive care units have, at one time or another, "septic work-ups," in which the blood, urine, and spinal fluid are examined for infection. If found, it is treated with antibiotics.

Hemolytic disease of the newborn

Red blood cells have surface markers, a type of "fingerprints" which characterize each individual. The most widely recognized markers are the ABO and Rh systems. There are many others which are less familiar but nonetheless important. If the markers of the mother and fetus are different, the blood cells of the fetus may gain entry into the mother's circulation, where they induce an antibody response. If subsequent fetuses have the same markers, the antibodies from the mother may pass through the placenta and into the fetus, where they attack the red blood cells and break them down. Such a sequence of events may result in varying degrees of anemia and jaundice in the newborn period. One of the best known and most serious types of hemolytic disease relates to the Rh system. The ABO and other blood group systems may result in significant, but less severe, anemia and jaundice.

Low blood sugar (hypoglycemia)

The brain and heart are highly dependent upon adequate amounts of sugar. Preterm babies, growth-retarded babies, infants of diabetic mothers, and sick infants may have difficulty in maintaining appropriate blood sugar levels, making them particularly prone to brain damage due to hypoglycemia.

Seizures

Seizures do not constitute a disease; rather they are manifestations of some disease process. In the newborn they are ominous signs of two serious problems: (1) metabolic abnormalities (such as low blood sugar) or (2) injury to the brain caused by trauma or insufficient oxygen. Seizures are treated by correction of the metabolic disturbance (if it exists) and by anticonvulsants.

Intravenous feeding (hyperalimentation, total parenteral nutrition)

This is a process of administering complete nutrients directly into the bloodstream. Very premature infants, very sick infants, or infants who have had intestinal tract surgery may not tolerate oral feedings, which ordinarily provide adequate nutrition for growth and recovery from illness.

Infants of diabetic mothers

While these babies are not born with diabetes, they may undergo stress during pregnancy due to the complications associated with diabetes in the mother (such as kidney problems and inadequate control of blood sugar). Some studies suggest a higher incidence of congenital birth defects (congenital heart disease, for example) in this group than in the population as a whole. Infants of diabetic mothers are more likely to be large, although preterm; as newborns, they are likely to have significant difficulties in maintaining normal blood sugars.

THE EFFECTS OF PERINATAL INJURY ON FUTURE DEVELOPMENT

In the early 1960s, Great Britain established perinatal risk registers in order to determine what effects unfavorable perinatal events might have on future development. The predictive validity of such registers has been inconsistent, varying with the criteria for inclusion in the high-risk groups. The literature on the subject is extensive, and there are many areas of controversy and confusion.

In 1979, Nelson and Ellenberg studied forty thousand infants and reported on signs of neonatal neurologic dysfunction which were predictive of future motor dysfunction.* Increases in the risk of cerebral palsy were observed in children with any one of the characteristics on the following page.

---

*K. B. Nelson, & J. H. Ellenberg. Neonatal signs as predictors of cerebral palsy. **Pediatrics,** 1979, *64*, 225.

FACTORS ASSOCIATED WITH INCREASED RISK

Factor	Relative risk
Overall impression of abnormality of brain function by the attending physician	99†
Neonatal seizures	71
Apgar scores of three or less at ten minutes or later	54
Multiple apneic episodes	36
Need for nasogastric feedings	22
Head circumference three standard deviations above or below the mean	21-26
Five-minute Apgar scores of three or less	21
Diminished activity or diminished crying lasting more than one day	19-21
Birth weight less than 2,000 gr.	16
Thermal instability	13
Hypertonia or hypotonia	12-15
Bilirubin equal to or greater than 20 mg./100 ml.	12
Hematocrit less than 40 percent	11

†That is, children with apparent brain dysfunction at birth are 99 times more likely than other children to have or develop cerebral palsy.

When an older child has significant developmental problems, it is not unusual to find that there were complications in the perinatal period. On the other hand, many children who have complications in the newborn period turn out to be normal, and many children with cerebral palsy had no problems as newborns. Further work is needed to define those events or combinations of events which predict unfavorable outcomes so that identification resources can be focused on these high-risk groups

SEE ALSO

Cerebral Palsy, Low Birth Weight, and *Respiratory Distress Syndrome*

Phenylketonuria and Other Metabolic Diseases

Frederick R. Schultz, M.D.

Phenylketonuria

DESCRIPTION

Phenylketonuria (PKU) is one of the best-studied inherited errors of body metabolism. Untreated PKU almost always results in severe mental retardation; it may also cause convulsions, behavior problems, severe skin rash, and a musty odor of the body and urine. With early diagnosis and appropriate treatment, all these manifestations of the disease can be prevented.

CAUSE

PKU results from the body's inability to convert phenylalanine, an essential amino acid found in high-protein foods, to another amino acid called tyrosine. This conversion, which takes place in the liver, depends on the presence of the enzyme phenylalanine hydroxylase. Children with PKU do not have this enzyme, and as a result the phenylalanine level in their body tissues becomes markedly elevated. Phenylalanine is then converted to phenylketones by a little-used chemical process. (The excretion of phenylketones in the urine is what led to the name "phenylketonuria.") It has been presumed—though never proven in laboratory experiments—that the very elevated levels of phenylalanine (or one of its by-products) are toxic to the body's tissues and therefore cause the clinical features of PKU.

For a child to inherit PKU, both parents must be carriers. That is, while neither parent has the clinical features of PKU, both have one gene for PKU, and both pass it on to the child. (There are, at present, no completely reliable laboratory tests to detect carriers.)

INCIDENCE

PKU occurs in approximately one in ten thousand to one in twenty thousand live births, depending on the ethnic background of the population. It is higher among groups of European ancestry. When both parents are carriers, the chances of having a child with PKU are one in four with each pregnancy.

DETECTION

Since 1964, mass screening of newborn infants has been adopted by most states and many foreign countries. A drop of blood is taken from the child's heel just prior to hospital discharge. If the blood test shows elevated levels of phenylalanine, the test is repeated for confirmation. Diagnosis must be prompt, since treatment should begin as soon after birth as possible.

COURSE

Left untreated in the first few months of life, PKU can lead to severe mental retardation and serious behavior problems. Formerly, many persons with PKU lived in residential institutions. Today, with appropriate diagnosis and dietary treatment, children with PKU can grow and develop normally.

ACCOMPANYING HEALTH PROBLEMS

Children with appropriately diagnosed and treated PKU are as active and healthy as children without PKU. However, women with PKU—treated or untreated—are at increased risk for bearing children with microcephaly, congenital heart disease, and mental retardation. Presumably these impairments result from the high levels of phenylalanine to which their babies are exposed during pregnancy. There is some speculation that in the future these abnormalities may be prevented by restricting the mother's phenylalanine intake prior to conception and during pregnancy.

MEDICAL MANAGEMENT

Once the diagnosis of PKU is confirmed, the infant is put on a special phenylalanine-restricted diet. It is important that the child's dietician be experienced in dietary treatment of children with PKU. Most of the caloric intake is in the form of a special formula (e.g., Lofenalac or

Phenyl-Free), from which nearly all the phenylalanine has been removed. A certain amount of phenylalanine must be added to the diet, however, to allow for normal growth. As the child becomes older, limited amounts of cereals, fruits, and vegetables are usually permitted. Meats, dairy products, and other high-protein foods are prohibited because of their high-phenylalanine content. (The formula provides most of the dietary protein.) Blood phenylalanine levels must be monitored frequently so that necessary adjustments can be made in the diet. PKU clinics have different policies regarding how long a phenylalanine-restricted diet should be continued. Most clinics recommend it for at least the first six years of life. Some clinics recommend allowing the children to eat a normal diet after age six; other clinics permit a wider variety of foods but continue some restriction of phenylalanine; still other clinics continue the phenylalanine-restricted diet. Many clinics have found it difficult to ensure strict adherence to the diet when the child reaches school age.

IMPLICATIONS FOR EDUCATION

Provided children with PKU are appropriately diagnosed and treated with a phenylalanine-restricted diet, they are no different from normal, healthy children and should be treated accordingly. There is no evidence of motor, perceptual, language, or attentional problems which interfere with the educational process. Symptoms of illness will be unrelated to the PKU and should be dealt with according to normal procedures. Nearly all children with PKU who are in early education programs will be following a phenylalanine-restricted diet. It is essential that educators communicate with parents to ensure the child's compliance with the crucial dietary treatment.

Other Metabolic Diseases

Early detection is important for a number of other metabolic disorders, including congenital hypothyroidism, galactosemia, and branched-chain ketoaciduria. Like PKU, these conditions can be screened for in the newborn period. Positive test results should be confirmed immediately, since infants with galactosemia and branched-chain ketoaciduria can become seriously ill in the first week of life, with a substantial risk of death or long-term disability. Also, since all the conditions screened for can produce brain damage, it is well to begin treatment as early as possible.

CONGENITAL HYPOTHYROIDISM

With this metabolic disease, the thyroid glands fail to develop normally. As a result, there is little or no thyroid hormone, a substance necessary for normal growth and development in childhood. This condition, which affects one in five thousand newborns, occurs sporadically and is not inherited from parents.

Children who are hypothyroid during early infancy have poor growth and little appetite. They are also sluggish and constipated. As newborns, they are likely to have jaundice, large protruding tongues, and poor muscle tone, with resultant umbilical hernias. Not every child with congenital hypothyroidism has these signs and symptoms, however.

With proper treatment, children with congenital hypothyroidism are healthy and without serious medical problems. Prior to newborn metabolic screening, many children with this condition were not detected early enough for treatment to be effective. Generally speaking, if significant mental impairment is to be prevented, treatment with replacement thyroid hormone must begin in the first three months of life. Children who began treatment with thyroid hormone before three months of age have shown normal intellectual functioning at five years. Their continued long-term functioning is also expected to be normal.

GALACTOSEMIA

This condition occurs with an absence of the liver enzyme galactose-l-phosphate-uridyl transferase. Without this enzyme, galactose reaches high levels in the blood and tissues, with resultant liver disease, kidney disease, blindness (due to cataracts), and mental retardation.

Galactosemia, which occurs in one in every fifty thousand births, is passed on through autosomal recessive inheritance. That is, both parents must be carriers of a gene for the disease. At present, many clinics are recommending that women who have previously given birth to children with galactosemia undergo amniocentesis. If the fetus has galactosemia and the pregnancy is continued, the mother may be advised to restrict her intake of galactose during the latter part of pregnancy.

Children with galactosemia are treated with a special diet free of galactose (a substance found in both human and cow's milk). They are generally given one of the soy-based formulas (Isomil, Neo-Mull-Soy, Nursoy). Later, as they grow older and begin eating solid foods, they must avoid foods containing milk or milk products. Children treated early with a galactose-free diet are generally healthy and able to avoid serious medical problems. Whether early treatment results in completely normal intellectual ability and overall functioning, however, remains to be fully documented.

BRANCHED-CHAIN KETOACIDURIA

Children with branched-chain ketoaciduria (maple syrup urine disease) are unable to metabolize three amino acids—namely, valine, leucine, and isoleucine. This is a very rare condition, occurring in only one in every one hundred fifty thousand births; both parents must be carriers of a gene which causes it.

Affected chidren are fed a specially manufactured formula from which valine, leucine, and isoleucine have been removed. Since these three amino acids are essential for growth and development, small amounts of regular milk are given as a supplement. As the children begin eating solids, foods containing protein are prohibited or introduced only in small, carefully measured quantities. At the present time it is recommended that children with branched-chain ketoaciduria continue on a protein-restricted diet throughout childhood and into adulthood.

Although early treatment of branched-chain ketoaciduria has certainly reduced medical problems, there is as yet insufficient data to predict how early treatment of this disease will affect intellectual capabilities and overall functioning in adult life.

Children with branched-chain ketoaciduria may become suddenly and seriously ill with what in normal children would be a mild viral illness, such as a cold or stomach flu. They may then require further modification of their diet or possibly artificial removal (peritoneal dialysis) of the branched-chain amino acids valine, leucine, and isoleucine (and the products of their metabolism) from body tissues. It is important that these children be treated at a medical center with experience in the management of branched-chain ketoaciduria.

SEE ALSO

Genetics

Positioning and Handling

Loretta Knutson Lough, L.P.T., M.A.

Positioning

Positioning is the process of placing a child with developmental disabilities in adapted or specially designed equipment to facilitate better posture and performance.

WHY POSITION A CHILD WITH DISABILITIES?

Standard, unadapted child care equipment often does not provide the necessary postural support for the individual with developmental disabilities. Lacking normal control of the body, the child may lean to one side, arch the back, or fall forward. Over extended periods, this may lead to joint contractures, scoliosis, hip dislocations, and other structural problems. Poor positioning can also cause pressure sores (decubitus ulcers).

Poorly Positioned Child—
Note leaning to one side.

Properly Positioned Child

The child who is properly positioned in adapted or specially designed equipment is more comfortable, may perform better, and has less chance of developing deformities. Proper positioning has advantages for the caretaker as well, making the child easier to feed, transport, and otherwise manage.

EVALUATING THE CHILD'S POSITIONING NEEDS

Because body alignment can affect the whole spectrum of a child's learning and development, a team of professionals is usually involved in evaluating the child prior to ordering adaptive equipment: typically, **(1)** physical and occupational therapists determine motor and adaptive function levels; **(2)** a nurse or physician evaluates general health status;

(3) a speech pathologist reviews language comprehension and speech motor skills; (4) a psychologist measures social and intellectual abilities; (5) a teacher determines educational goals; (6) an audiologist assesses hearing; and (7) a social worker identifies individual family needs—which *must* be considered if the equipment is to be put to proper use. When these evaluations are completed and reviewed by team members, the physical and occupational therapists are ready to measure the child and to select, order, and fit the appropriate equipment.

POSITIONING EQUIPMENT

Maintaining the best possible position for everyday functioning may include (1) adapting available childcare equipment, such as a stroller, carseat, highchair, potty chair, or classroom chair; (2) utilizing therapeutic equipment, such as a wheelchair; or (3) constructing equipment from original designs. While such equipment is usually for sitting, devices are also used for side lying, standing, and other positions. Depending on the needs of the individual, adaptive equipment may have inserts for maintaining specific angles and inclines as well as head and neck supports and appropriate restraining straps.

THE IMPORTANCE OF FOLLOW-UP

A child needs to build up skin or behavioral tolerance to the adapted equipment gradually. A specific program for increasing tolerance is recommended. Once positioning is completed, the child should be reevaluated and the equipment examined at regular intervals. Changes in growth and motor abilities often require changes in the adaptive device.

Handling

The child with a neuromuscular disorder must be picked up and carried correctly.

INCORRECT—Avoid lifting the child under the arms without supporting the legs. The child with high muscle tone (hypertonicity) may "scissor" the legs. The child with low muscle tone (hypotonicity) may slip through your hands.

CORRECT—Bend the child's legs before picking her up. Provide good support for both the trunk and legs. Encouraging rotation in the trunk is good, particularly for the child with high muscle tone.

Gather the child with low muscle tone close to you to give him a feeling of stability.

For distances, you may want to have the child straddle your hip.

SEE ALSO

Bracing, Cerebral Palsy, and *Myelomeningocele*

Respiratory Distress Syndrome

Frederick R. Schultz, M.D.

DESCRIPTION

Respiratory distress syndrome (RDS) is a pulmonary disorder commonly encountered in premature infants. It is among the most frequent causes of death in the premature infant as well as the most common illness in many neonatal intensive care units. The usual signs are labored, grunting respirations, poor oxygenation of body tissues in room air, and characteristic findings on chest X-ray examinations.

CAUSE

Respiratory distress syndrome is caused by a deficiency of a material called surfactant, which is needed to keep the air sacs (alveoli) in the lungs open. When surfactant is absent or when it is present in inadequate amounts, the air sacs, and hence the entire lung, collapses (a condition known as atelectasis). The tremendous energy which is then required to breathe leads to exhaustion and the above-mentioned signs of RDS.

A fetus seldom produces adequate amounts of surfactant before 36 weeks gestation. RDS is therefore common among premature infants. This condition rarely occurs in full-term infants unless the lungs are particularly immature, as they may be, for example, in infants born to women with diabetes.

INCIDENCE

RDS occurs in 1 percent of newborns, making it the most common severe respiratory problem in the first few days after birth. The incidence of RDS varies greatly with gestational age; it is rare in full-term infants and extremely common in infants born prior to 32 weeks gestation.

DETECTION

Generally speaking, respiratory distress syndrome is not difficult to detect clinically. Usually within a few hours after birth, the premature baby audibly grunts on expiration, breathing frequently and with great effort, flaring the nostrils and retracting the muscles between the ribs and just below the rib cage. The infant is also lethargic and has a bluish color due to decreased oxygen concentration in the blood.

COURSE

Depending on the prematurity of the infant, the duration of RDS may be one to two days, or it may last more than a week. This condition usually improves when the infant begins producing adequate amounts of surfactant.

ACCOMPANYING HEALTH PROBLEMS

Premature infants suffering from respiratory distress syndrome are vulnerable to other health problems associated with prematurity. One of the most important of these is bleeding into the fluid-filled spaces of the brain (intraventricular hemorrhage), a condition often associated with later disabilities.

Infants with very severe respiratory distress syndrome, especially those who are on a mechanical ventilator for prolonged periods or those who receive high concentrations of oxygen, are at risk for developing a chronic lung disorder known as bronchopulmonary dysplasia (BPD).

MEDICAL MANAGEMENT

Neonatal intensive care units, anticipating RDS in premature infants, routinely monitor pulse and respiration, along with the amount of oxygen in the blood. At the first clinical sign of RDS, treatment is begun. This may initially take the form of increasing the concentration of inspired oxygen. Often, constant distending pressure through the nose or mouth (continuous positive airway pressure, or CPAP) is applied to keep the alveoli and lungs from collapsing. Some infants require a mechanical ventilator, which essentially breathes for them. Infants with RDS usually are not able to nurse or drink formula from a bottle; they must either be fed intravenously or given formula or breast milk through a tube which is passed through the mouth or nose and into the stomach.

IMPLICATIONS FOR EDUCATION

Today, approximately 90 percent of infants with RDS survive. Of these, the majority will develop normally and do well in regular classes. A small group, however, particularly those who have experienced intraventricular hemorrhage or other medical complications during the early days of life, may have developmental disabilities which include cognitive and/or physical impairment. Some may have continuing problems with respiratory illness, especially during the first year. Breathing difficulties, cough, or fever should always be evaluated by a health provider.

SEE ALSO

Low Birth Weight

Routine Health Care

James A. Blackman, M.D.

When children are receiving care and treatment for developmental disabilities or impairments, routine health care may be neglected. This is especially problematic for two reasons: **(1)** handicapped children may be more prone to certain common illnesses, such as colds, ear infections, or diarrhea, and **(2)** with these children it is often more difficult—though particularly important—to distinguish routine illnesses from more serious ones.

SCHEDULE OF PREVENTIVE HEALTH CARE RECOMMENDED BY THE AMERICAN ACADEMY OF PEDIATRICS

AGE	INFANCY						EARLY CHILDHOOD					LATE CHILDHOOD					ADOLESCENCE			
	By 1 mo.	2 mos.	4 mos.	6 mos.	9 mos.	12 mos.	15 mos.	18 mos.	24 mos.	3 yrs.	4 yrs.	5 yrs.	6 yrs.	8 yrs.	10 yrs.	12 yrs.	14 yrs.	16 yrs.	18 yrs.	20 yrs.
HISTORY Initial/Interval	•	•	•	•	•	•	•	•	•	•	•	•	•	•	•	•	•	•	•	•
MEASUREMENTS Height and Weight	•	•	•	•	•	•	•	•	•	•	•	•	•	•	•	•	•	•	•	•
Head Circumference	•	•	•	•	•	•	•	•												
Blood Pressure										•	•	•	•	•	•	•	•	•	•	•
SENSORY SCREENING Vision	S	S	S	S	S	S	S	S	S	O	O	O	O	O	S	O	O	S	O	S
Hearing	S	S	S	S	S	S	S	S	S	S	S	S	S	S	S	S	S	S	O	S
DEVEL./BEHAV. ASSESSMENT	•	•	•	•	•	•	•	•	•	•	•	•	•	•	•	•	•	•	•	•
PHYSICAL EXAMINATION	•	•	•	•	•	•	•	•	•	•	•	•	•	•	•	•	•	•	•	•
PROCEDURES Hered./Metabolic Screening	•																			
Immunization		•	•	•		•	•				•						•			
Tuberculin Test	↓								•		↑	↓		•		↑	↓		•	↑
Hematocrit or Hemoglobin	↓				•				•		↑	↓		•		↑	↓		•	↑
Urinalysis	↓			•					•		↑	↓		•		↑	↓		•	↑
ANTICIPATORY GUIDANCE	•	•	•	•	•	•	•	•	•	•	•	•	•	•	•	•	•	•	•	•
INITIAL DENTAL REFERRAL										•										

Any suspected problems should be promptly investigated regardless of the child's age.

Children with disabilities should be seen by a dentist within six months from the eruption of the first tooth.

THE HEALTH CARE PROVIDER

It is essential that every child be seen regularly by a health care provider. This is especially true of a child with disabilities, since chronic disease, poor nutrition, and medications all influence developmental progress. Also, any leveling off or regression in development may be a sign of specific neurological disease. Therefore, although most handicapped children are involved with developmental assessment and treatment agencies, it is important that the primary health care provider keep abreast of the child's developmental progress as well.

One important function of the primary health care provider is to counsel parents regarding proper diet, including adequate calorie intake as well as a proper balance of protein, fats, and carbohydrates. This medical professional should also teach parents how to monitor their child's health and recognize early signs of illness, including:

- Change in personality or habits
- Fever
- Change in appetite
- Change in bowel or urinary habits
- Irritability
- Lethargy
- Vomiting
- Diarrhea

The primary health care provider should also counsel parents on how a disability may affect their child's behavior and development. Otherwise, misunderstandings may occur. For example, a behavior syndrome that is caused by hypersensitivity to environmental stimuli—a result of central nervous system damage—may be mistaken for prolonged, severe colic. Likewise, the sudden and abnormal rigidity in infants suffering from spasticity may be misconstrued by anxious parents as rejection.

In addition to counseling parents, the primary health care provider should advise other professionals on the child's health limitations as well as on how to recognize new or recurrent health problems. This physician—the pediatrician or general practitioner—should also facilitate communications among parents, medical subspecialists, and nonmedical professionals. It is the primary health care provider with whom the education-related professional should discuss both the child's general health and specific disability-related concerns.

SEE ALSO

Dental Disease and *Growth and Nutrition*

Seizure Disorders

Mark L. Wolraich, M.D.

DESCRIPTION

Seizures, also called convulsions, are characterized by involuntary motor activity or a change in consciousness or behavior. These are symptoms of underlying abnormalities of the brain. Normally, minute electrical impulses travel along specific nerve pathways in a controlled fashion and at appropriate times. A seizure occurs when bursts of unorganized electrical impulses interfere with this normal brain functioning. Electrical bursts of different types or in different locations of the brain result in different kinds of seizures. Epilepsy is a chronic condition of the nervous system that is characterized by recurrent seizures.

Grand mal seizures

These seizures, which account for 60 percent of all convulsive disorders, are generalized throughout the body. Prior to onset of a grand mal seizure, the child may experience a very brief warning, or aura; this can take the form of numbness, noise, taste, smell, or other unusual sensations or feelings. The seizure itself has two phases: tonic and clonic. During the tonic phase there is usually loss of consciousness, stiffening of the body, heavy and irregular breathing, drooling, skin pallor, and occasional bladder and bowel incontinence. After a few seconds, the clonic phase begins. The clonic phase is characterized by alternating rigidity and relaxation of the muscles. The tonic and clonic phases are usually followed by a period of drowsiness, disorientation, or fatigue (the postictal state).

Focal seizures

Focal seizures are caused by abnormal electrical impulses in a localized area of the brain. This can occur in the motor strip of the right frontal lobe, for example, in which case there may be involuntary, repetitive jerking of the left hand and arm.

Focal seizures may become generalized and result in loss of consciousness.

Infantile spasms

Also called infantile myoclonic seizures or jacknife epilepsy, infantile spasms usually begin when a child is three to nine months old. Episodes, characterized by dropping of the head and flexion of the arms, may occur hundreds of times a day. The developmental prognosis of infants with this type of seizure is generally (though not always) poor; while the spasms may abate after several years, other types of seizure may replace them. Infantile spasms may indicate the presence of an underlying disorder, such as tuberous sclerosis. They are associated with a typical EEG pattern called hypsarrhythmia.

Myoclonic-akinetic seizures

Myoclonic seizures, not to be confused with infantile myoclonic seizures (see above), are characterized by brief, involuntary jerking of the extremities, with or without loss of consciousness. Akinetic seizures, on the contrary, are characterized by loss of tone. These two types of seizure may be related to fixed neurological damage or to a degenerative process. They are often very difficult to control.

Psychomotor seizures

Sometimes referred to as temporal lobe seizures, this type is caused by abnormal electrical bursts in the temporal lobe of the brain. It is usually characterized by involuntary, repetitive behaviors, such as chewing, lip smacking, or rubbing of the hands or legs. Affected individuals may have unusual sensory experiences or undergo emotional changes, becoming fearful or angry. The seizure may last from a few seconds to a few minutes—with the child in an altered state of consciousness. It is commonly followed by confusion.

Petit mal seizures

Petit mal seizures occur most commonly between the ages of four and twelve years and usually disappear as the child reaches maturity. About one-third to one-half of the individuals who have petit mal seizures will also have (or eventually develop) grand mal seizures. Petit mal seizures are more difficult to recognize: the child usually appears to be staring absentmindedly, sometimes repetitively blinking the eyes or smacking the lips. The episodes are brief, usually lasting from 5 to 30 seconds. There is loss of consciousness without loss of muscle tone; this means that the child does not fall down yet has no memory of the episode and is unaware of the passage of time.

Simple febrile seizures

Perhaps the most common type of seizure—occurring in 5 to 10 percent of children under the age of five—is one that is precipitated by fever. This type of seizure, which typically lasts less than ten minutes, tends to occur during a febrile illness in a child between the ages of one and six. It is characterized by loss of consciousness and involuntary, generalized jerking. (It is, in fact, a grand mal seizure.)

There is some controversy about whether or not to treat children with febrile seizures; most physicians, however, feel it is not necessary to treat the child who has only one uncomplicated febrile seizure. The vast majority of children who have simple febrile seizures are not harmed by them and do not develop epilepsy. However, children who have focal or prolonged febrile seizures and children who have a history of abnormal development or abnormal findings on a neurologic exam are at increased risk for developing epilepsy.

CAUSE

The reasons for seizures are as varied as the types. In most cases the cause in unknown; that is, the seizure is idiopathic. At times, it is possible to identify a hereditary component. Also, any injury to the brain can bring about a seizure disorder. A severe head injury or brain hemorrhage can cause scarring in the brain, where abnormal bursts of electricity may originate. Scarring can also be caused by meningitis or encephalitis or by congenital infections, such as rubella. Other conditions associated with seizures include cerebral palsy, hydrocephalus, and metabolic disorders.

INCIDENCE

Seizure disorders occur in 0.5 percent of the general population.

DETECTION

Most seizures are easy to detect because of their obvious clinical manifestations. However, psychomotor and petit mal seizures can sometimes have atypical clinical signs which make the diagnosis more difficult.

When seizures have occurred, a brain wave test (electroencephalogram, or EEG) is usually obtained. Electrodes placed on different areas of the scalp record the electrical impulses caused by the brain activity. In most circumstances, the EEG provides helpful confirming evidence of a seizure disorder. For example, if a grand mal seizure is coupled with a characteristic pattern on the EEG, the physician has a clear diagnosis. The EEG alone, however, is not sufficient to diagnose a seizure disorder. The seizure disorder may not show up in the EEG pattern, or the EEG pattern may be abnormal when there is no clinical evidence of seizures.

Children with petit mal seizures and infants with infantile myoclonic seizures both have a very specific disorganized pattern on their EEGs. EEG patterns do not always correlate with clinical seizure types, however. In some instances the location rather than the pattern of abnormal electrical discharges can be significant. For instance, children with psychomotor seizures show an abnormal EEG in those electrodes which are placed over the temporal lobe region of the brain.

COURSE

Without anticonvulsant medications, most children with seizure disorders will have recurrences of seizures. In the majority of cases—particularly with grand mal, focal, petit mal, and psychomotor seizures—anticonvulsants can prevent recurrence once the appropriate dosage requirement has been determined—provided the child receives the medication regularly. With some children, however, seizures are not easily controlled; they may require multiple changes in medications and dosage. With a few children, it is impossible to totally control seizures. While this can be true of any type of seizure disorder, it is more frequently the case with myoclonic or mixed seizure disorders or when there is severe brain damage or severe mental retardation.

Seizures may disappear or decrease in frequency as the child gets older, but it sometimes happens that one type of seizure is replaced by another type (e.g., infantile spasms may be replaced by grand mal seizures). There can be a recurrence of, or increase in, seizure activity around puberty, when hormonal changes may inhibit the brain's ability to restrict the abnormal bursts of electricity. Many times, after a number of years have gone by without a seizure—and provided there is no cause to suspect a continuing disorder—physicians will try taking children off anticonvulsants to see whether seizures will recur.

ACCOMPANYING HEALTH PROBLEMS

Seizure disorders frequently accompany other disorders, including cerebral palsy, myelomeningocele, encephalitis and meningitis, and mental retardation.

ANTICONVULSANT MEDICATIONS
AND THEIR SIDE EFFECTS

Name	Type of seizures treated	Side effects/ adverse reactions
Carbamazepine (Tegretol)	Grand mal Focal Psychomotor	Vomiting, headache, drowsiness, blood dyscrasia, ataxia
Clonazepam (Clonopin)	Petit mal Myoclonic (Minor motor)	Hyperactivity, short attention span, impulsive behavior, drowsiness, ataxia, vertigo or dizziness, confusion, excessive weight gain, drooling
Corticosteroids ACTH	Infantile myoclonic	Moon face, elevated blood sugar, susceptibility to infections, thinning of the bones, muscle weakness
Diphenylhydantoin (Dilantin)	Grand mal Psychomotor Focal	Gingival hyperplasia, hirsutism, dermatitis rash (in approximately 5-10 percent of patients; drug should be discontinued), drowsiness, gastric distress, nystagmus, ataxia, dysarthria, blood dyscrasias
Ethosuximide (Zarontin)	Petit mal	Dizziness, GI distress: nausea, vomiting, anorexia; leukopenia, kidney dysfunction
Phenobarbital (Luminal)	Grand mal	Rash (Stevens-Johnson syndrome), ataxia, hyperactivity, questionable effect on cognitive performance, blood dyscrasias
Primidone (Mysoline)	Grand mal Psychomotor	Drowsiness, dizziness, abnormal behavior, ataxia, rash, blood dyscrasias, diplopia, nystagmus
Valproic acid (Depakene)	Petit mal Grand mal Mixed myoclonic-akinetic	Nausea, vomiting, drowsiness, incoordination, dizziness, skin rash, liver toxicity, hair loss, weight gain

MEDICAL MANAGEMENT

Seizure disorders are treated with anticonvulsant medications. The two most commonly used medications are phenobarbital and phenytoin (Dilantin). These are the first-line medications for grand mal seizures. If they are not effective, carbamazepine (Tegretol), primidone (Mysoline), or valproic acid (Depakene) may be added. Ethosuximide (Zarontin) is used with petit mal seizures, carbamazepine and primidone with psychomotor seizures, and clonazepam (Clonopin) with myoclonic seizures. Anticonvulsants are frequently ineffective with infantile myoclonic seizures, and both steroids and ACTH (a hormone secreted by the pituitary gland) have been tried with varying degrees of success.

Uncomplicated seizure disorders are frequently managed by pediatricians and family physicians. More complex cases, however, require consultation with a neurologist. Ongoing follow-up is required because seizures can change in intensity and type with time. The medication and dosage also need to be checked as the child grows. Also, the child should be monitored for adverse side effects.

IMPLICATIONS FOR EDUCATION

Grand mal seizures in and of themselves usually are not harmful unless they are very prolonged or recur in rapid succession (*status epilepticus*), in which cases immediate medical care is needed. Otherwise, the main concern is that the child does not become injured from falling. During the seizure, breathing is frequently irregular. It may even appear to stop, but this is rarely the case. Usually, the only first aid required is preventing self harm. It is best to keep the child on his or her side to prevent food from getting into the lungs should vomiting occur. Contrary to popular notions, it is *not* necessary to prevent the child from swallowing the tongue. In fact, trying to put something in the mouth can result in the loss of the child's teeth or injury to the first aid provider's fingers. In the rare case where breathing has actually stopped, as might occur if regurgitated stomach contents are aspirated, standard cardiopulmonary resuscitation (CPR) techniques should be employed immediately.

Both a poorly controlled seizure disorder and the side effects of many of the anticonvulsant medications can affect alertness and academic performance. Changes in behavior should be reported to the child's physician. It is also important for teachers to take note of the child's behavior just prior to and during a seizure and to report this as well.

FIRST AID
· FOR EPILEPTIC SEIZURES

A major epileptic seizure is often dramatic and frightening. It lasts only a few minutes, however, and does not require expert care. These simple procedures should be followed:

- **REMAIN CALM.** You cannot stop a seizure once it has started. Let the seizure run its course. Do not try to revive the child.

- If the child is upright, ease him to the floor and loosen his clothing.

- Try to prevent the child from striking his head or body against any hard, sharp, or hot objects; but do not otherwise interfere with his movement.

- Turn the child's face to the side so that saliva can flow out of his mouth.

- **DO NOT INSERT ANYTHING BETWEEN THE CHILD'S TEETH.**

- Do not be alarmed if the child seems to stop breathing momentarily.

- After the movements stop and the child is relaxed, allow him to sleep or rest if he wishes.

- It isn't generally necessary to call a doctor unless the attack is followed almost immediately by another seizure or the seizure lasts more than ten minutes.

- Notify the child's parents or guardians that a seizure has occurred.

- After a seizure, many people can carry on as before. If, after resting, the child seems groggy, confused, or weak, it may be a good idea to accompany him home.

Courtesy of:
EPILEPSY FOUNDATION OF AMERICA

SEE ALSO
Electroencephalography

Teratogens

David P. Schor, M.D.

Teratogens are agents in the environment of the developing embryo and fetus which cause structural or functional abnormalities. About 8 percent of birth defects are clearly linked to teratogens. The percentage of birth defects due to teratogens may actually be much higher, however, since the causes of most congenital anomalies are unknown.

Causes of Developmental Defects in Man—Estimates Based on Surveys and Case Reports in the Medical Literature

Known genetic transmission		20%
Chromosomal aberration		3-5%
Environmental causes		
Ionizing radiations		<1%
Therapeutic	Nuclear	
Infections		2-3%
Rubella virus	Varicella virus (?)	
Cytomegalovirus	Toxoplasma	
Herpes virus hominis	Syphilis	
Maternal metabolic imbalance		1-2%
Endemic cretinism	Phenylketonuria	
Diabetes	Virilizing tumors	
Drugs and environmental chemicals		4-5%
Androgenic hormone	Anticonvulsants	
Folic antagonists	Oral hypoglycemics(?)	
Thalidomide	Few neurotropic-anorectics(?)	
Oral anticoagulants	Organic mercury	
Maternal alcoholism		
Combinations and interactions		?
Unknown		65-70%

Source: Wilson, :J. G., & Frazer, C. (Eds.). *The handbook of teratology* (Vol. 1). New York: Plenum Press.

Several factors interact to determine the occurrence and severity of a teratogenic effect. Among them are the timing of exposure (stage of pregnancy), the genetic makeup of the fertilized egg, genetic and environmental factors in the mother, and the type and dosage of the teratogen itself. The time at which susceptibility to damage is greatest varies with the different developing organ systems. In general, exposure during the first two weeks of pregnancy either results in spontaneous abortion or has no effect at all. Exposure during weeks three through seven is likely to result in the abnormal growth and development of a body part. Later exposure may produce disturbances in the *functioning* of certain organs though their general *structure* appears normal.

Schematic illustration of the sensitive or critical periods in human development. The dark band indicates stages that are less sensitive to teratogens. Note that each organ or structure has a critical period during which its development may be deranged, and that physiological defects, functional disturbances, and minor morphological changes are likely to result from disturbances during the fetal period. Severe mental retardation may result from exposure of the developing human to high levels of radiation during the 8- to 16-week period.

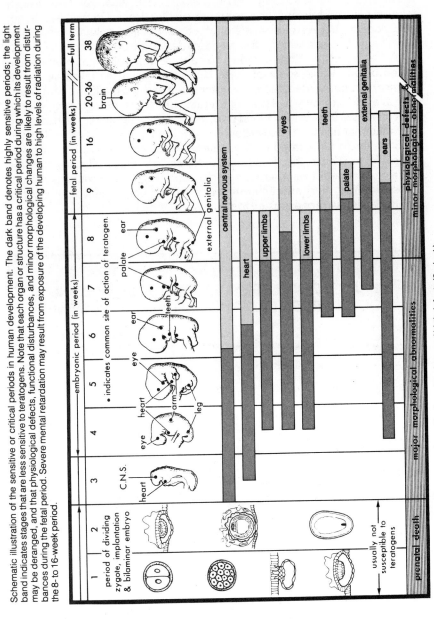

Source: Moore, K. L. *Before we are born: Basic embryology and birth defects* (2nd ed.). Philadelphia: W. B. Saunders.

Substances may be teratogenic for some animals and not for others. While many drugs and chemicals have resulted in birth defects when administered to animals in large doses, it is not certain what significance such studies have for humans receiving much smaller doses. On the other hand, thalidomide, believed to be safe on the basis of initial animal studies, was later found to cause abnormal arm and leg development in humans.

A few agents which are known to cause abnormalities in humans are listed below. While some of these high-risk substances (alcohol, for instance) can be avoided, there are situations in which it is difficult or impossible to avoid exposure to a potential teratogenic agent. For example, a drug to control seizures or high blood pressure may be teratogenic yet necessary for maternal health; if medication is discontinued, the fetus as well as the mother could be harmed by the maternal disorder. While it is sometimes possible to reduce the dosage or to switch to equally effective but less teratogenic medicines, there are instances in which such changes are not possible. Also, there are circumstances in which neither the woman nor her physician is aware of exposure to a known teratogen.

EXAMPLES OF AGENTS CAPABLE OF CAUSING DEVELOPMENTAL ABNORMALITIES IN HUMANS

Class	Example	Common effect	Time of maximum chance of harm	Chance of harm
Radiation (high doses)	Radiotherapy	Mental retardation Small head Skeletal abnormalities	First ⅓ of pregnancy	High
Infection	Rubella (German measles)	Cataracts Congenital heart disease Deafness	First 5 weeks of pregnancy	15-20 percent
Maternal metabolic imbalance (untreated)	Phenyl-ketonuria	Mental retardation Congenital heart disease	Unknown	95 percent
Drugs and environmental chemicals	Ethanol (alcohol)	Small head Mental retardation Poor growth	Unknown	Unknown

Visual Impairment

David P. Schor, M.D.

While newborns can see quite well, a normal adult level of visual acuity is not present at birth; rather, it develops gradually and depends upon proper functioning of all structures of the visual system. For normal vision to occur, images must be accurately transmitted to the brain, as illustrated below:

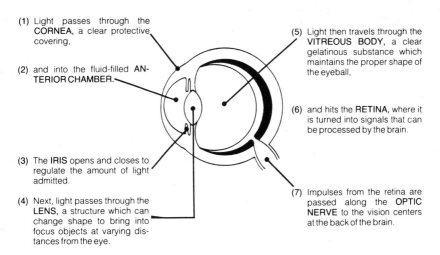

(1) Light passes through the **CORNEA**, a clear protective covering,

(2) and into the fluid-filled **ANTERIOR CHAMBER.**

(3) The **IRIS** opens and closes to regulate the amount of light admitted.

(4) Next, light passes through the **LENS**, a structure which can change shape to bring into focus objects at varying distances from the eye.

(5) Light then travels through the **VITREOUS BODY**, a clear gelatinous substance which maintains the proper shape of the eyeball,

(6) and hits the **RETINA**, where it is turned into signals that can be processed by the brain.

(7) Impulses from the retina are passed along the **OPTIC NERVE** to the vision centers at the back of the brain.

How Light Is Transmitted to the Brain

Primary visual impairment may arise from problems at any step in this process. Also, improper image reception during infancy can result in secondary—and often permanent—abnormalities.

CAUSES

Light is blocked from the retina

Sometimes the structures that normally transmit light from the eye surface to the retina—the cornea, anterior chamber, lens, and vitreous body—act instead to block the image. Abnormalities in one or more of these structures result from exposure during pregnancy or birth to certain viruses or bacteria, from chemical eye burns or eye trauma, or from increased pressure within the eye which is present at birth (congenital glaucoma). In some cases, a clouding of the lens (cataract) accompanies certain infections or inherited disorders, such as rubella or Down syndrome.

Images are not focused on the retina

Vision is also impaired if the image is not focused clearly on the retina. This occurs with nearsightedness (myopia), farsightedness (hyperopia), and uneven focusing of the image on the retina (astigmatism).

Nearsightedness

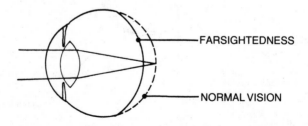

Farsightedness

Nerve impulses are blocked from reaching the brain

Disorders which can block the path of nerve impulses from the retina to the vision centers of the brain include tumors of the retina, brain injury, and retrolental fibroplasia. (Retrolental fibroplasia is a disease of the retina which occurs in some premature infants who required oxygen for treatment of respiratory distress. Mild cases may resolve completely without visual impairment. More severe cases, however, may result in retinal damage and loss of vision. Retrolental fibroplasia may be accompanied by strabismus and refractive errors.)

The brain fails to process information from the eyes

Some children may have problems with "central processing" of visual information. That is, the structures which transmit visual information to the brain are intact, but the information reaching the brain is not processed or interpreted in a meaningful way. This may occur in children with damage to the visual cortex in the occipital lobes or in children with generalized cerebral dysfunction which produces significant intellectual defects.

Strabismus

With this condition, sometimes called "squint," the eyes do not work together. One eye may consistently turn inward (or outward), or the eyes may alternate in their deviation from proper alignment. Strabismus may result from weakness of the muscles which control eye movement, from ocular defects such as cataracts or a damaged retina, or from poor visual acuity.

Since sensory input is necessary for proper development of the visual system, untreated stabismus may result in further loss of functional vision. Therefore, infants who continue to show signs of strabismus by six months of age are referred to an ophthalmologist for evaluation. In every case, the most important goal of treatment is to preserve the best possible vision. If possible, the underlying cause is treated. With poor visual acuity, for example, cataracts are removed or glasses are prescribed. At times, a child may be forced to use the weaker eye by patching the normal eye. Occasionally, surgery may be necessary to correct alignment.

INCIDENCE

Blindness occurs in about one in four thousand children. Less severe yet significant visual defects occur in about one child in 20. The rate of visual impairment is much higher among children with multiple handicaps; one study found significant visual abnormalities in 30 percent of multiply handicapped children whose primary diagnosis did not involve vision.

DETECTION

Screening for actual or potential visual abnormalities in children is important. During infancy or early childhood—the optimal time for preventing or minimizing visual impairments—most children are not aware (or cannot communicate) that their vision is faulty. A child's eyes should be examined for abnormalities and muscle imbalance at birth, at 3, 6, and 12 months, and annually thereafter. At these intervals the parents should be asked whether they have noticed the child crossing the eyes, holding objects close to the face, failing to focus on faces or objects, exhibiting poor eye-hand coordination, or performing any other acts which suggest possible visual problems.

Visual acuity testing becomes more precise as the child develops. With various commonly used tests, preschool children may be asked to name objects (STYCAR) or pictures (Allen), or to point in the direction of the "legs" of the letter E. Children under 12 months may be observed as they track brightly colored objects. Another method of assessing vision in very young children or in children with significant developmental delays uses an electroencephalogram (EEG) in combination with a computer to assess the brain's response to specific visual stimuli, such as a flashing light. These responses (called visual evoked responses, or VER) are compared with those of children who have normal vision.

While vision screening is important for all children, it is especially valuable for those with a history of visual problems or for those who have had certain infections around the time of birth. Other events, such as exposure to prolonged supplemental oxygen following premature birth, are serious enough to warrant an examination during the first few months of life by an ophthalmologist, a physician with specialized training in disorders of vision.

MEDICAL MANAGEMENT

Most children, even those who are very young, may wear glasses. Only young children, however, can strengthen the muscles in one eye by wearing a patch over the other. Surgery may be necessary to treat cataracts, glaucoma, or, in older children, uncorrected strabismus.

Poor eyesight has been blamed for certain learning problems, especially reading disabilities. The American Academy of Ophthalmology, however, has found the incidence and spectrum of learning problems to be the same among children with and without learning disabilities. This organization is very skeptical about the benefits of eye muscle and visual tracking exercises and other so-called visual training techniques in the treatment of learning and other developmental problems.

IMPLICATIONS FOR EDUCATION

Because visual impairment is common and rarely produces signs or symptoms readily traceable to the visual system, children must have regular vision system assessments. At high risk for vision problems are children with disabilities, children who were born prematurely or who suffered intrauterine growth retardation, and children with family histories of visual impairment. Early detection, combined with appropriate referral and effective treatment, can significantly improve vision among affected children.

Frequent squinting, rubbing of the eyes, lack of attention, or irritability may be associated with visual problems and should be reported to the child's parents.

Whenever possible, the activities and experiences of children with visual impairment should be accompanied by verbal expression and tactile interactions.

SEE ALSO

Cerebral Palsy, Congenital Infections, and *Low Birth Weight*

Helpful References

Batshaw, M. L. & Perret, Y. M. *Children with handicaps: A medical primer.* Baltimore: Paul H. Brookes, 1981.

Bleck, E. E. & Nagel, D. A. (Eds.). *Physically handicapped children: A medical atlas for teachers.* New York: Grune and Stratton, 1975.

Gadow, K. D. *Children on Medication: A primer for school personnel.* Reston: The Council for Exceptional Children, 1979.

Halsam, R. H. A. & Valletutti, P. J. (Eds.). *Medical problems in the classroom: The teacher's role in diagnosis and management.* Baltimore: University Park Press, 1975.

Peterson, R. M. & Cleveland, J. O. *Medical problems in the classroom: An educator's guide.* Springfield: Charles C. Thomas, 1975.

Special Interest Organizations

American Foundation for the Blind, Inc.
15 West 16th Street
New York, New York 10011

Cystic Fibrosis Foundation
6000 Executive Boulevard, Suite 309
Rockville, Maryland 20852

Down's Syndrome Congress
528 Ashland Avenue
River Forest, Illinois 60305

Epilepsy Foundation of America
1828 L Street, Suite 405
Washington, D.C. 20036

Muscular Dystrophy Association, Inc.
810 Seventh Avenue
New York, New York 10019

National Association for Down's Syndrome
Box 63
Oak Park, Illinois 60303

National Association for Retarded Citizens
2709 Avenue E East
P.O. Box 6109
Arlington, Texas 76011

National Association for the Visually
  Handicapped
305 East 24th Street, Room 17-C
New York, New York 10010

National Association of the Deaf
814 Thayer Avenue
Silver Spring, Maryland 20910

National Association of the Deaf-Blind
2703 Forest Oak Circle
Norman, Oklahoma 73701

National Association of the Physically
  Handicapped
76 Elm Street
London, Ohio 43140

National Center for a Barrier-Free
  Environment
1140 Connecticut Avenue, Suite 1006
Washington, D.C. 20036

National Easter Seal Society for
  Crippled Children and Adults
2023 West Ogden Avenue
Chicago, Illinois 60612

National Federation of the Blind
1346 Connecticut Avenue N.W.
Suite 212, Dupont Circle Building
Washington, D.C. 20036

National Paraplegia Foundation
333 North Michigan Avenue
Chicago, Illinois 60601

National Society for Autistic Children
1234 Massachusetts Avenue N.W.
Suite 1017
Washington, D.C. 20005

Spina Bifida Association of America
343 South Dearborn Street, Room 317
Chicago, Illinois 60604

United Cerebral Palsy Associations, Inc.
66 East 34th Street
New York, New York 10016

Taken from:

Clearinghouse on the Handicapped, Office for Handicapped Individuals, Office of Human Development, U.S. Department of Health, Education, and Welfare. *Directory of National Information Sources on Handicapping Conditions and Related Services.* Washington, D.C.: Author, 1976.

Index